KU-780-856

CONTENTS

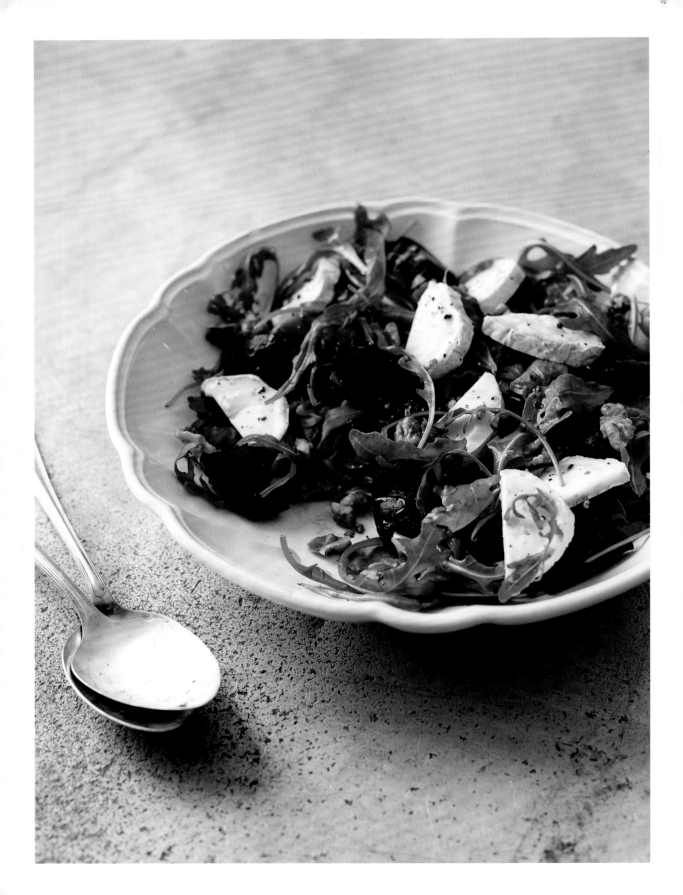

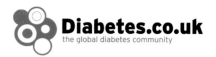

Diabetes.co.uk
the global diabetes community

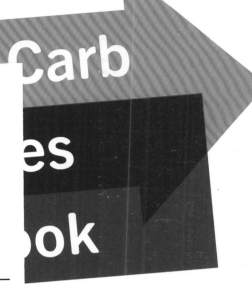

The Low-Carb
...es
...ook

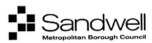

Sandwell
Metropolitan Borough Council

Please return this item to any Sandwell Library on or before
the return date.

You may renew the item unless it has been reserved by
another borrower.

You can renew your library items by using the 24/7 renewal
hotline number - 0845 352 4949
or FREE online at opac-lib.sandwell.gov.uk

THANK YOU FOR USING YOUR LIBRARY

HA
31/7/19

...) help control
...2 diabetes

...MMA PORTER

Vermilion

12888458

10 9 8 7 6 5 4 3 2 1

Vermilion, an imprint of Ebury Publishing,
20 Vauxhall Bridge Road,
London, SW1V 2SA

Vermilion is part of the Penguin Random House group of companies whose
addresses can be found at global.penguinrandomhouse.com

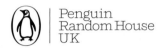
Penguin
Random House
UK

Copyright © David Cavan 2018, Emma Porter 2018 and Diabetes Digital
Media Limited 2018

David Cavan and Emma Porter have asserted their right to be identified
as the authors of this Work in accordance with the Copyright, Designs
and Patents Act 1988

Photography: Kim Lightbody
Food Styling: Becci Woods
Design: Maru Studio
Project Management: Laura Nickoll

First published by Vermilion in 2018

www.penguin.co.uk

A CIP catalogue record for this book is available from the British Library

ISBN: 9781785041402

Printed and bound in China by C&C Offset Printing Co., Ltd

All rights reserved. No part of this publication may be reproduced, stored in
a retrieval system or transmitted, in any form or by any means, electronic,
mechanical, photocopying, recording or otherwise, without the prior
permission of the publishers.

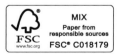

Penguin Random House is committed to a sustainable
future for our business, our readers and our planet.
This book is made from Forest Stewardship Council®
certified paper.

The information in this book has been compiled by way of general guidance
in relation to the specific subjects addressed, but is not a substitute and not
to be relied on for medical, healthcare, pharmaceutical or other professional
advice on specific circumstances and in specific locations. So far as the authors
are aware the information given is correct and up to date as at June 2018.
Practice, laws and regulations all change, and the reader should obtain up
to date professional advice on any such issues. The authors and publishers
disclaim, as far as the law allows, any liability arising directly or indirectly
from the use, or misuse, of the information contained in this book.

Foreword

BY DR DAVID CAVAN

As a consultant specialising in diabetes, it is fair to say that for most of my career, I focused on advising medication first and foremost as the means to help people achieve good control of their diabetes. And yet in so many cases, without success. Then, less than ten years ago, I actually started to focus in detail on what my patients were eating, and realised that the officially recommended low-fat, high-carbohydrate diet was a big part of the problem, contributing to excess weight gain and poor diabetes control. I therefore started to advise a low-carbohydrate, healthy fat diet, as outlined in my book, *Reverse your Diabetes: the Step by Step Plan to Take Control of Type 2 Diabetes*.

Following its publication, I very soon started receiving reports from people who had adopted the recommended diet and seen great improvements in their weight and their diabetes control. Many were able to come off medication and some were successful in reversing their diabetes.

However, the benefits of such a diet are not just confined to those with type 2 diabetes. Given that highly refined carbohydrates contribute to the development of type 2 diabetes, it is extremely effective for people with prediabetes, to help prevent them progressing to developing 'full-blown' type 2 diabetes, and for those who are gaining weight and at risk of prediabetes in the future. It is also effective in enabling people with type 1 diabetes to achieve stable glucose control on less insulin, which means less risk of hypos and less risk of unwanted weight gain.

It has therefore been a great pleasure to team up with Emma Porter, a successful food writer who herself has type 1 diabetes, in writing this book. Not only has she compiled some great and healthy recipes, her experience of living with diabetes and with the impact of how food affects glucose control brings a welcome and unique credibility.

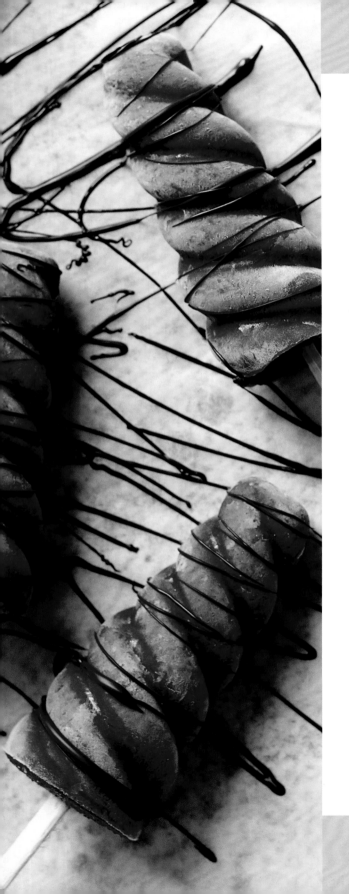

Foreword

BY EMMA PORTER

AS A TYPE 1 DIABETIC, I spent a lot of my younger years trying to be 'normal' by largely ignoring my diagnosis: drinking and eating what I wanted and behaving just like my non-diabetic friends.

I was young, naive – and newly diagnosed. I was bullied in my early teens causing me to comfort eat, and although I never had an unhealthy relationship with food, I used chocolate as a comforter, as a soothing, kind friend that helped ease my sadness and loneliness.

Following my diagnosis I was constantly misinformed by the medical profession about what I should and shouldn't eat. Repeatedly doctors and nutritionists told me that I should consume a low-fat, high-carb diet and drink diet drinks. I followed this lifestyle for years and experienced only a constant blood sugar rollercoaster while never really understanding WHY. When, all along, the simple answer was the food I was eating.

In my mid-twenties, I took hold of the reins of my disease. Contrary to the dietary advice I was being given, I decided on a low-carb approach. I realised that the only person who could change and make things better for me was me. I cooked every single meal, I got up earlier to eat breakfast or I prepared it the night before. I made things like frittatas (page 52) to take with me to work as snacks and the results were pretty instant. I started sharing the food I was making on social media and my blog and people started to follow me. They tried the dishes I was making and the feedback was truly astonishing.

Over the last four years there has been a lot of development and fine tuning. My husband is my greatest fan and supporter. He has been my loyal and very willing guinea pig. Luckily for me he is a big foodie, having grown up in a pub, so I can trust his comments and suggestions. My daughter, who was born in 2016 and is now a toddler, is one of my biggest inspirations and is now another of my guinea pigs! It is of paramount importance to me that she understands where food comes from and has a healthy relationship with food, without relying heavily on sugar or processed foods.

Food for me should be simple to make, an enjoyable experience, not cause arguments, taste delicious and be there for everyone to savour. I want people to WANT to go back for seconds, and I want the recipes to be shared. Life is too short not to eat nice food.

These days, there are too many weird 'superfood' ingredients that cost a small fortune and usually end up sitting in your cupboard. Green powders that are meant to change your life, but quite frankly taste like gone-off pond water. The recipes in this book are all based on readily available ingredients, no special equipment beyond what you would find in most kitchens and require only modest culinary skills. But they are all about REAL food. No powders, no absurdly expensive hard-to-find ingredients, just a regular shopping list.

Of course all food is 'real' food. What I mean is food that has not been processed. Food that doesn't have dozens of additives and hidden ingredients. Food that doesn't come from the freezer section, a takeaway or in a packet promising things like 'eat this and you'll lose weight'. Food that is cooked from scratch with natural, unprocessed ingredients.

Be open-minded and try new things. If you don't like a certain ingredient in a recipe then change it to something similar, but obviously be realistic! Eating low carb isn't about eating bland, boring and tasteless foods. It isn't about being on a restrictive 'diet'. Try the recipes and you will find that eating low carb can be a delicious, health-altering lifestyle choice.

I have always loved cooking and experimenting with taste, flavour and texture. I used to spend my summers working in pubs, saving as much money as I could to travel to wonderful and inspiring places. Places where simple, fresh ingredients are the basis of any delicious dish and where carbs are not a staple or vital to the meal.

So when it came to writing the recipes for this book, I wanted to communicate my passion for simple, well-balanced, tasty recipes that can be enjoyed by the whole family, including the kids. Whether you are type 1, type 2 or a non-diabetic, these low-carb, blood sugar-friendly recipes should benefit everyone.

What has happened to our food?

Our eating habits have changed enormously over the past 30 years. However, these changes have been quite subtle and gradual, so that until someone points them out to you, you might not have noticed them.

The majority of these changes started in the 1970s and many people under the age of 40 will be even less aware of what has happened. As I am well over 40, I can remember the food environment in the 1970s (and the 1960s) and can see how different it is today.

These changes have been brought about by a number of factors, including:

In the 1970s
• Nutrition guidelines promoted a low-fat diet.
• Changes in agriculture promoted low-cost grains and sugar byproducts (such as high-fructose corn syrup) developed as sweeteners for many foods and drinks.
• The wider availability of home freezers, meaning that large quantities of food could now be stored, including, for the first time, ice cream.
• Supermarkets began to sell a wide range of processed and frozen foods.

In the 1980s
• The arrival of microwave ovens prompted a new market in 'ready meals'.
• Expansion of fast-food outlets, selling high-calorie foods at cheap prices.

In the 1990s
• Coffee shops appearing on high streets, selling more high-calorie foods and drinks, in an inviting environment that commanded more expensive prices.
• The growth of supersize portions, which encouraged us to eat and drink more than we needed, duping us into believing we were getting a bargain.

And driving the changes throughout this period was a global food industry that has grown exponentially and has used various media avenues to market their products to an unsuspecting public.

The effect of all these changes, and more, has been to turn us from the society we were in the 1970s to today's society. Then, most meals were eaten in the home, prepared from fresh natural ingredients bought in season from local shops and sweets, ice cream, crisps and fizzy drinks were an occasional treat and usually eaten outside of the home. Today, we eat 'on the hoof' – at fast-food restaurants, coffee shops or other outlets

– with far fewer meals being eaten at home. In addition, many of those meals eaten at home are bought ready-made (and, by definition, processed) and not prepared at home from fresh ingredients.

Many products bought in supermarkets have been processed to remove fat and add sugar, so that foods that naturally contain fat, such as dairy products, can now claim to be low fat and thus 'healthy'. And foods that used to be an occasional treat, such as sweets, ice creams, crisps and fizzy drinks have now become part of our everyday diet.

At the same time that all this has been happening, food has become ever more plentiful and cheaper. In the 1970s food was, in real terms, more expensive than it is now, and that is particularly the case for unhealthy foods. For example, a packet of crisps is much cheaper in major supermarkets than a single apple. While eating out used to be an expensive occasional event, fast snack-type food is now available everywhere. Whenever I travel to London by train and arrive at a main station I now have to resist the temptations of several outlets selling all manner of high-calorie foods, whereas in the 1970s there was just one rather uninspiring cafeteria to greet me.

It is the same story on our high streets, where fast-food chains and coffee shops are in abundance. Thinking about these changes isn't just a case of nostalgia, but rather it should help us understand how dramatically our modern environment has changed since the days up until the Second World War, when hunger was prevalent, and how, without much in the way of countering forces, this new way of eating has inadvertently but inevitably encouraged the spread of obesity.

Taken together, these changes mean there has been a transformation in our food environment. Put simply, we have access to a whole variety of foods and drinks that were just not available 30 or 40 years ago.

Throughout history, our ancestors have eaten the food that is most readily available to them. That is why Inuits ate fish and whale fat, and bushmen in Africa ate vegetables and meat. Modern man is no different, but what has changed is that the food we are surrounded by is unnatural, very high in sugars and processed fats and in many countries is readily available in high quantities and at low prices. As if that wasn't bad enough, many foods and drinks have been manufactured by an industry more interested in profit than our health, and that uses marketing techniques to tempt us into buying inherently unhealthy foods. Many of these foods have quasi-addictive properties and can be used (or abused) for comfort.

I guess that throughout history our ancestors didn't necessarily analyse everything they ate – they simply ate what was available, and it is the same now. So our current unhealthy eating patterns have just become accepted. That chocolate bar that you buy at the service station, the muffin with your coffee, the can of Coke and packet of crisps with your lunch – these are now so common as part of our everyday routine, that, by definition, they have become normal.

Yet over that same period of time we have become less healthy, more of us are now overweight or obese, and more people are developing type 2 diabetes. We now know there is a direct link between our food and our health. Most of the foods that we eat to excess are characterised by high levels of sugar or other refined carbohydrates. These stimulate the body to produce high levels of insulin, causing a condition known as hyperinsulinaemia (high insulin in the blood). Insulin is the body's main fat-storage hormone, so hyperinsulinaemia is associated with increased body weight and increased fat stores in the liver and other organs. It also directly contributes to high blood pressure and high cholesterol levels, as we will explore in the next chapter.

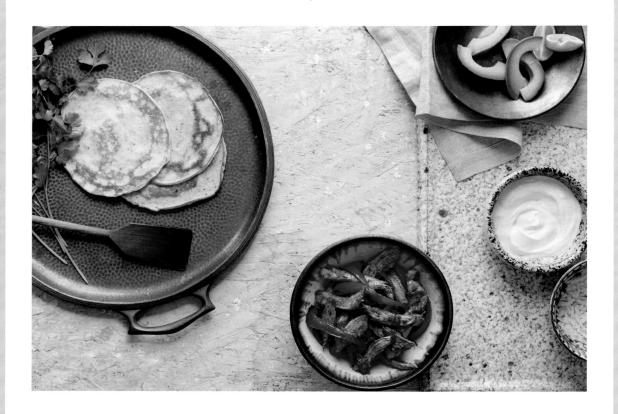

What unhealthy food does to us

OBESITY AND TYPE 2 DIABETES

In the 40 years since we were advised to follow a low-fat diet, the rates of type 2 diabetes have increased in almost every country in the world. In 2017, the International Diabetes Federation estimated that 425 million adults were living with diabetes, and that over 90 per cent of these were cases of type 2 diabetes.

Type 2 diabetes is a condition where the level of glucose in the bloodstream is higher than normal. It usually occurs from middle age onwards, but increasingly it is being seen in younger people. Its onset is usually gradual, without any specific symptoms, and sometimes it is first diagnosed by a screening blood test. However, if left untreated, rising blood glucose levels lead to symptoms such as excessive urination, increased thirst, tiredness, blurred vision and weight loss, as well as infections such as thrush.

These symptoms arise because in diabetes glucose cannot enter the body's cells and so it accumulates in the bloodstream. As glucose is not getting into the body's cells, they are starved of energy, which leads to weight loss and tiredness. As the blood glucose level rises, the kidneys try to excrete the excess glucose in the urine. This explains why glucose can be detected in the urine. Its sugary nature provides an ideal environment for the growth of bacteria and fungi, which leads to urinary infections and thrush (candidiasis). In order to excrete glucose the kidneys need to excrete a larger volume of water (otherwise you would be peeing out sugar lumps) and this leads to dehydration, which in turn leads to excessive thirst. High glucose levels in the eyes leads to blurred vision.

Over the longer term, high glucose levels can cause damage to small blood vessels throughout the body, which can lead to the long-term complications of type 2 diabetes. These include damage to the retina in the eye, to the kidneys and nerves, and an increased risk of heart attack and stroke. Good control of blood glucose greatly reduces the risk of these complications. Type 2 diabetes is best controlled by lifestyle changes, principally by modifying diet. However, many people are prescribed drugs to control type 2 diabetes, and until relatively recently it was thought that most people with the condition would eventually need insulin.

THE ROLE OF INSULIN IN KEEPING GLUCOSE LEVELS UNDER CONTROL

In order to understand why glucose levels rise in people with type 2 diabetes, it is important to understand how insulin controls glucose levels when everything is working normally. Glucose is a type of sugar that is used for energy by nearly all types of cells in the body, so it is essential that all parts of the body have a steady supply of it. This glucose is obtained from the food we eat: the carbohydrates (sugars and starch) that we consume are broken down into glucose, which is then absorbed from the gut into the bloodstream so that it can be carried to all tissues and used as energy. Any spare glucose is taken up into the muscles and liver, where it is stored in the form of glycogen. Glycogen in the muscles is then available for later use if the muscles need extra energy (for example, during intensive exercise). Once the glycogen stores are full, any excess glucose is converted to fat and stored in the liver.

While glucose only enters the body when we eat or drink, the body's cells require a constant supply of it in order to function properly. The liver, which releases some of its stored glucose into the bloodstream, provides this service and ensures that just the right amount of glucose is available during periods when we are not eating (for example, overnight). In a person who does not have diabetes, the amount of glucose in the bloodstream is maintained at around 4–6mmol per litre (or 80–120mg per decilitre.)

The level of glucose in the bloodstream is controlled by insulin.

Insulin is a hormone that is produced by the pancreas, which is an organ that sits just below the rib cage, behind the stomach. The pancreas has two main functions. One is to produce enzymes that are released directly into the small intestine, which break down food so it can be absorbed into the bloodstream. These enzymes include amylase, which breaks down starch into glucose; lipase, which breaks down fat; and protease, which breaks down proteins.

The other main function of the pancreas is to produce hormones. These are chemicals that are released into the bloodstream and which have effects all around the body. Insulin is one of the hormones produced by the pancreas and, as already mentioned, its job is to regulate the level of glucose in the bloodstream, ensuring that cells get the right amount at all times. It does this in a number of ways:

1. When we eat a meal the carbohydrate it contains is converted into glucose in the gut and passes through the gut wall into the bloodstream. The body detects that the glucose level in the blood is rising and this leads to the pancreas producing additional insulin.

2. This insulin acts on individual cells to allow glucose to enter them. Insulin molecules attach to a receptor on the cell membrane that opens up to allow glucose in. Insulin is often likened to a 'key' that opens the cell's 'door', allowing glucose to enter it.

3. Insulin also stops the liver and muscles from releasing stored glucose into the

bloodstream; this allows spare glucose to be added to the glycogen stores.

4. When we are not eating, the pancreas continually produces a small amount of insulin that controls the release of glucose from the liver. In the liver insulin acts like a tap that turns off the release of glucose from the liver. If glucose levels in the blood drop too low, less insulin will be produced (opening the tap), allowing more glucose to be released from the liver. On the other hand, if glucose levels rise, more insulin is produced, closing the tap and slowing down the release of glucose from the liver.

The main problem in type 2 diabetes is that insulin doesn't work very well; this reduced effectiveness interferes with both the action of insulin in turning off the tap that releases glucose stored in the liver into the bloodstream, and its role in opening the cell doors to allow glucose to enter the body's cells after a meal.

It seems that the problem starts in the liver, which becomes 'immune' or resistant to the effect of insulin so that even when insulin is present the liver keeps releasing glucose into the bloodstream. This is called 'insulin resistance', and to try to get round this the pancreas produces more and more insulin in an attempt to control the release of glucose from the liver. For a while this may work in keeping the blood glucose level under control, but eventually the liver becomes resistant to even these high levels of insulin and so the level of glucose in the blood rises. Diabetes develops once the blood glucose

rises above a certain level – that is, above 7mmol per litre (126mg per decilitre) if fasting, or above 11.1mmol per litre (200mg per decilitre) after a meal.

Until the 1990s, type 2 diabetes was not readily associated with obesity. Certainly there were people who were obese and had type 2 diabetes, but there were also many people with type 2 diabetes who, while a little overweight, were not obese at diagnosis. However, over the past 20 years there has been a steady increase in the number of people diagnosed with type 2 diabetes. There has also been quite a sharp increase in the number of people who are overweight or obese. In the 1990s, it was estimated there were 1 million people in the UK with diabetes, the majority of whom had type 2 diabetes. By 2017 this had increased to around 3.7 million – and it is estimated that over 30 per cent of the population were obese.

In 2014, it was reported that rates of type 2 diabetes had reached 29 million in the US, or 9.1 per cent of all adults in the country. That's not to mention the millions estimated to have undiagnosed type 2 diabetes. Rates of obesity, meanwhile, have more than doubled since 1980; in 2009–10 data showed that 35.7 per cent of American adults were obese. And while by no means all cases of type 2 diabetes are caused by obesity, there is certainly a distinct correlation between the two conditions.

This has led to a big shift in the way we think about the disease. It is now abundantly clear that in many cases type 2 diabetes has developed in individuals as a result of their being overweight.

The message is now very clear: if you eat too much you will become overweight. And if you become overweight there is a greatly increased chance of developing type 2 diabetes. The bad news is that on an individual level this means there is a direct link between a person's lifestyle and later development of type 2 diabetes; the good news is that this readily explains why lifestyle changes can help control diabetes – and raises the possibility that changing lifestyle might help reverse the condition.

Thus, if you are overweight and/or have type 2 diabetes, your eating habits are likely to have played a role in causing it. However, it would not be right to blame yourself entirely for having become overweight or developing type 2 diabetes. Remember that this is a problem affecting millions of people across the world, which has come about as a result of the changes in food production and processing that have brought about an unhealthy food environment, while other lifestyle changes have made us less physically active.

FAT IN THE LIVER

If we consume more than we need the human body is very efficient at storing the excess energy as fat. We all know that if we put on weight we become a bit chubbier due to increased fat tissue below the skin. This is what causes a double (or triple) chin, for example. We also know that men in particular are prone to carrying fat around the middle, the so-called beer belly. This fat is in the abdominal cavity and surrounds organs such as the gut. With the advent of body scanning it has become apparent that many people who are overweight develop what is termed fatty liver, which is just that – excess fat deposited in the liver itself.

We have known for some time that people with fatty liver may show evidence that their liver function is affected, not in a dangerous way, but enough to show up on blood tests where the levels of liver enzymes, such as alanine aminotransferase (ALT) are raised. Occasionally fatty liver can progress to cirrhosis, which is associated with permanent scarring of, and damage to, the liver. Research published in 2011 suggested that this excess fat in the liver is very significant in the development of diabetes, as it is the excess fat that makes the liver resistant to insulin. This means that insulin can no longer stop glucose leaving the liver and entering the bloodstream (the insulin 'tap' becomes leaky, letting glucose levels rise in the blood). In order to compensate for this the pancreas produces more insulin. However, one of the effects of high insulin levels is that even more fat is then deposited in the liver, which in turn makes the problem even worse. Over time not only does the liver become filled with fat, but so too does the pancreas. And just as a liver full of fat cannot work properly, a pancreas that is filled with fat can no longer produce insulin normally; recent evidence suggests that less than one gram of extra fat in the pancreas is enough to affect insulin production.

Although this theory may not explain every case of type 2 diabetes, it does explain how, in many people, obesity leads to diabetes – first by making the liver resistant to insulin, so that blood glucose levels rise, and then by affecting the pancreas so that it cannot produce insulin.

It also explains how some people of relatively normal weight may develop type 2 diabetes. Anyone whose diet leads to high insulin levels increases the likelihood of excess fat being deposited in the liver and so increases the risk of type 2 diabetes, even if they are not significantly overweight.

This is especially the case in many developing countries, where there has also been a big increase in rates of type 2 diabetes, but without the increase in obesity. It is also important to recognise that there are many people who are obese who do not have type 2 diabetes. It appears that people have different thresholds at which their bodies can tolerate the effect of too much fat in their internal organs. People with a lower threshold will develop type 2 diabetes sooner (and at a lower overall body weight) than those with a higher threshold. Nevertheless, insulin resistance is a common underlying factor behind both obesity and type 2 diabetes.

Having demonstrated how excess fat in the liver and pancreas leads to the development of type 2 diabetes, researchers examined the effect of sudden weight loss in people with established type 2 diabetes. They were asked to follow a strict 600-calorie per day liquid diet for eight weeks, with various blood tests and MRI scans done before and afterwards. The results were quite remarkable: within a week blood glucose levels returned to normal and this was accompanied by a big reduction in the amount of fat in the liver. Over the next few weeks the fat content in the pancreas also reduced. By eight weeks the pancreas was producing insulin normally and the liver was no longer resistant to the effect of insulin – the leaky tap had a new washer. Taken together these changes meant the people in the study no longer had type 2 diabetes.

These experiments confirmed the theory that type 2 diabetes is related to the amount of fat in the liver and in the pancreas. What was even more exciting was the discovery that a reduction in food intake could reverse the disease process. This is great news because it means that if you have recently been diagnosed with type 2 diabetes, by reducing your food intake and weight, there is a chance that you can become free from diabetes.

Further great news is that you do not have to adopt a very low-calorie diet to reverse type 2 diabetes. The same can be achieved by ensuring that the foods you eat do not cause big rises in your blood glucose level; this means your pancreas does not need to produce so much insulin; less insulin means less liver fat, less body weight and in some cases reversal of type 2 diabetes. These are the principles set out in my book *Reverse Your Diabetes: the Step by Step Plan to Take Control of Type 2 Diabetes* and it has been very heartening to hear from people who have put those principles into practice and successfully reversed their diabetes.

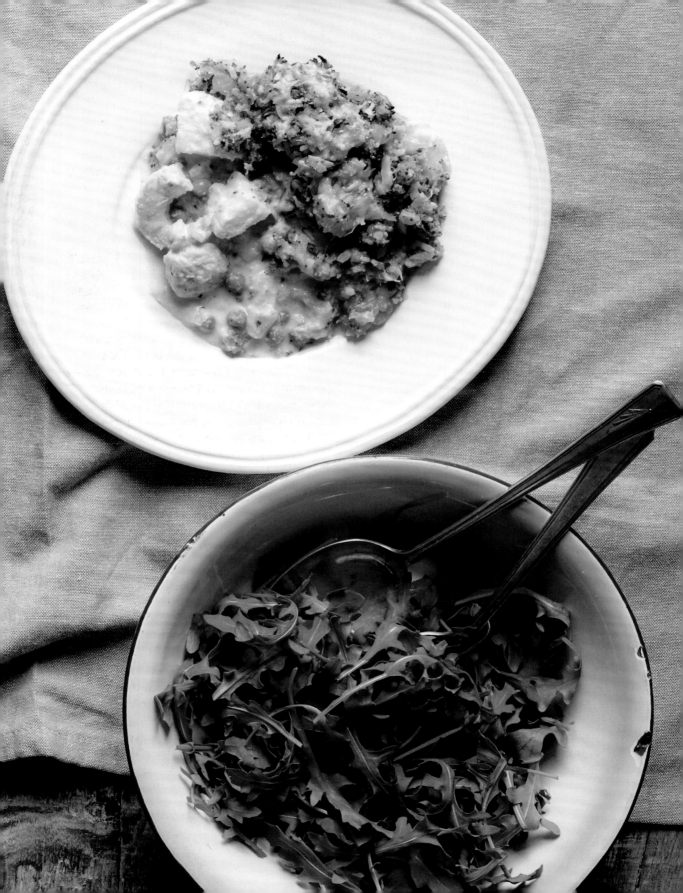

HIGH BLOOD PRESSURE AND HIGH CHOLESTEROL LEVELS

We have seen how type 2 diabetes and obesity result from the effects of insulin resistance and high insulin levels. Those same high insulin levels also contribute to high blood pressure and high cholesterol levels, and these are often also present in people with obesity or type 2 diabetes.

Blood pressure refers to the level of pressure that the blood is under in the blood vessels. The cells that make up the body need glucose and oxygen (plus a variety of other substances) to function effectively. The job of blood is to carry these necessary chemicals and nutrients to every part of the body. Blood is also the means by which hormones, produced in the pancreas and other endocrine organs, are transported to the different parts of the body, where they are needed to perform their biochemical action (in the case of insulin, enabling glucose to enter cells).

So for blood to function effectively it needs nice clean blood vessels to flow through and it needs to be under pressure in order to flow (against the force of gravity, a lot of the time). Obviously if there were no pressure the blood would just sit where it is, like a stagnant pool. Blood pressure comes primarily from the action of the heart, the specialised muscle that acts as a pump squeezing the blood through the arteries. The kidneys also have an important role in controlling blood pressure, both by regulating the amount of water in the blood vessels, and by producing hormones that help control how tightly the blood vessels contract (to increase pressure) or relax (to reduce blood pressure). It will be obvious that diseases of either the heart or the kidneys may cause problems with blood pressure regulation – and can make an existing blood pressure problem worse.

Blood pressure is reported as two numbers, for example 120/80. The first number is the pressure in the arteries as the heart is contracting (called systolic blood pressure) and the second number is the pressure as the heart is relaxing (called diastolic blood pressure).

So what should your blood pressure be? There are many guidelines that specify the ideal levels of blood pressure in different circumstances, but as a general rule it should be below 135/85. If you are young, or have evidence of kidney or eye disease, a lower level may be recommended. Here it is important to mention that blood pressure levels vary quite considerably during the day, according to what you are doing and experiencing. In fact, blood pressure can rise very quickly if, for example, you get a sudden shock or undertake sudden intense exercise or physical activity.

Being overweight and inactive are associated with hyperinsulinaemia, even in people who do not have type 2 diabetes. High insulin levels cause high blood pressure, because one of the functions of insulin is to retain sodium (salt) in the circulation. This is one of the reasons why people with insulin resistance, with or without type 2 diabetes, have high blood pressure.

A higher salt level in the body leads to more water remaining in the circulation, which, if excessive, can lead to high blood pressure. Now given that we are largely made up of salty water (or saline), it is clear that we need some salt in our diet. Indeed, people with too little salt can experience dizziness and fainting owing to their blood pressure being too low. However, many processed foods in our modern diet include far too much salt and if your blood pressure is high, reducing the salt in your diet can make a big difference. The first step is to try to avoid adding salt to your food at the table – pepper or other spices will add taste with no effect on your blood pressure. Then you should consider reducing the amount of salt you add during cooking. Obviously salt is important to enhance flavour, but not so much that you can actually taste the saltiness. However, the biggest challenge in reducing salt intake is knowing which foods contain it and in what amounts. Just about any savoury foods (and many sweet foods) that are not fresh will, in all likelihood, have salt added. And this not only includes highly processed foods (such as shop-bought, ready-made meals) that you may well perceive to be unhealthy anyway, but also more traditional foods such as bread, bacon and cheese. Sweet foods, such as breakfast cereals, may also contain salt. One reason that salt is used is to add flavour to low-quality ingredients therefore, you may find that cheaper, 'value' processed foods have a higher salt content than more expensive ones.

Just as hyperinsulinaemia has an effect on increasing blood pressure, it is also associated with overproduction of cholesterol in the liver and its release into the circulation. High cholesterol levels are also associated with an increased risk of heart attack and strokes. However, cholesterol has in my view been unfairly demonised. Let's be clear – the body needs cholesterol for many functions. Cell membranes, which control what enters into cells of the body, are largely made of cholesterol. Vitamin D, essential for healthy bones, and many hormones are also made from cholesterol. However, in today's society, too many of us have too much cholesterol in our bloodstream.

There are several types of cholesterol that have different actions. LDL-cholesterol is made in the liver and released into the bloodstream where, if too much is produced, it can be associated with narrowing of the arteries. HDL-cholesterol, on the other hand is good for you.

Now, some people have a high total cholesterol, but this is because there is a high level of healthy HDL. For this reason it is often easiest to look just at the LDL cholesterol when deciding if you need to make any changes. As with high blood pressure, there are no symptoms associated with having a high cholesterol level, and the only way to know if your cholesterol is raised is by having a blood test.

As with high blood pressure, the first thing to consider is whether there are any changes you can make to your lifestyle. And the good news is that exactly the same changes that will help reduce your blood pressure will also reduce your cholesterol level. So, increasing your physical activity, eating a healthy diet and losing weight will all contribute to reducing cholesterol levels. Beware of being taken in by low-fat foods, though. While there may seem to be a certain logic that says eating less fat will reduce your cholesterol level, remember that insulin is the main fat-producing hormone, and it is carbohydrates in your diet, and not fat, that increase insulin levels.

All this means that if you are able to make changes to your lifestyle that reduce insulin resistance – reducing insulin and glucose levels in your blood by reducing your intake of carbohydrates – then there is a good chance your cholesterol level and blood pressure will also come down, especially if and when you lose weight.

PREDIABETES

Prediabetes describes the situation in people whose blood glucose levels are higher than normal, but not yet high enough to be diagnosed as having type 2 diabetes. It is officially known as 'intermediate glucose tolerance' and is defined by a person having a fasting blood glucose between 5.5 and 6.9mmol

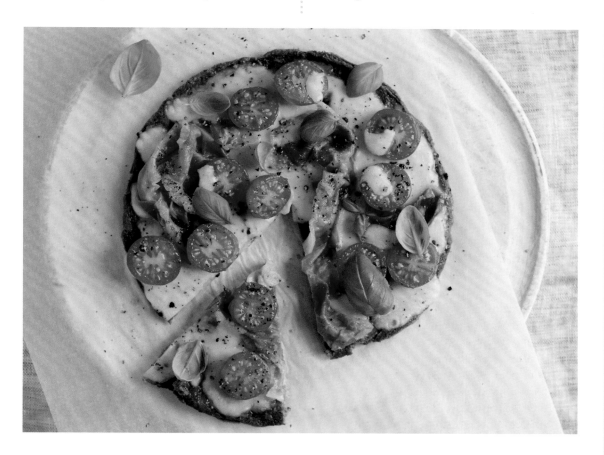

per litre (100–125 mg per decilitre) or a level between 7.8 and 11.1 mmol per litre (140 and 200mg per decilitre) two hours after having a drink containing 75 grams of glucose, as part of a diagnostic procedure called a glucose tolerance test. It is also diagnosed by an HbA1c blood test between 6 and 6.5 per cent (42–48 mmol/mol).

Prediabetes occurs in people who have become insulin resistant, but who are still able to maintain near-normal levels of glucose in their bloodstream. The bad news is that they are at high risk of progressing to type 2 diabetes; the positive news is that by making appropriate lifestyle changes, there is a good chance of not only halting the development of type 2 diabetes, but of reversing to normal. This has recently been demonstrated by Dr David Unwin, a family doctor from Southport, England. A few years ago, he started advising his patients with prediabetes to adopt a low-carbohydrate diet and showed that after an average of two years, over 90 per cent had reversed to normal glucose levels. This is a much greater success rate that was shown in the big diabetes prevention trials that used a low-fat diet.

POLYCYSTIC OVARY SYNDROME (PCOS)

This is a condition that is very common. The World Health Organization estimates that it affects over 3 per cent of women worldwide; other studies suggest that up to 18 per cent of women may be affected, many without having been diagnosed.

PCOS is usually diagnosed in young women and the main features are irregular or no periods, excess body or facial hair, having acne and being overweight or obese. In many cases the ovaries are found to contain many small cysts (hence the name), although these are the result of the condition, and not its cause. It is likely that the main cause is high insulin levels, that in affected women also impact the hormones that control the release of an egg (ovulation) each month and regular menstruation. These effects can result in infertility, weight gain and too much androgen (or male sex hormones) being produced, causing excess hair growth. Women with PCOS are at increased risk of developing type 2 diabetes in later life.

PCOS is usually diagnosed in young women in their teenage years or twenties. It is easy to understand how the problems it can cause can be very upsetting at this time of life. Treatments are directed at correcting the hormonal imbalance and encouraging weight loss. In my experience, many women with PCOS find it very difficult to lose weight, and I think this is for a number of reasons. In some cases, it can be because they don't feel very good about themselves, and such low self-esteem is a real barrier to making lifestyle changes; secondly, the effects of PCOS can often lead to a sense of depression, which itself can drive unhealthy 'comfort' eating. Finally, and perhaps most importantly, the high insulin levels actually make it very difficult for people to lose weight, especially if they follow a standard low-fat, high-carbohydrate diet that just stimulates yet more insulin to be produced.

Metformin (a treatment for type 2 diabetes that reduces insulin resistance) can be very effective in restoring regular periods and a low-glycaemic-index diet (i.e. avoiding highly refined carbohydrates) has also been shown to be beneficial. Individuals who are able to lose weight will often find that their periods (and their fertility) return as their hormones re-establish a normal balance.

TYPE 1 DIABETES

Unlike all the other conditions we have so far discussed, type 1 diabetes is not related to lifestyle but rather it is the result of the body's immune system attacking and destroying the cells in the pancreas that produce insulin. Like type 2 diabetes, people with type 1 diabetes have high glucose levels in the blood and are at risk of the same complications as a result.

Type 1 diabetes requires life-long treatment with insulin by injections or using an insulin pump. Although such treatment is life-saving, it is not the same as relying on insulin produced by the pancreas. A big difference is that injected insulin has to get from the place where it is injected (the fat below the skin) into the bloodstream and specifically to the circulation between the gut and the liver where it does most of its work. As a result, the levels of insulin in the general circulation are often much higher than in someone whose pancreas works normally. In other words, they have hyperinsulinaemia. Over time, these high insulin levels can lead to some of the problems we have discussed. These include weight gain and insulin resistance, that both mean a person needs to inject a higher dose of insulin to control their glucose levels. And that leads to even higher levels of insulin in the blood, more weight gain and potentially more insulin resistance, that in turn can aggravate high blood pressure and cholesterol levels. In other words, there is a risk of insulin treatment for type 1 diabetes causing problems similar to type 2 diabetes.

For most people with type 1 diabetes, the dose of insulin they inject depends on the amount of carbohydrate in their diet. Therefore, by reducing the carbohydrate in their diet, they are able to control blood glucose levels with lower insulin doses. Not only can this help people with type 1 diabetes lose weight, it can also greatly reduce the risk of blood glucose levels going too low (hypoglycaemia).

I have been recommending a low-carbohydrate diet for people with type 1 diabetes for some years and describe these principles in more detail in my book *Take Control of Type 1 Diabetes*.

EMMA: MY STORY

I was told I 'probably' had polycystic ovary syndrome (PCOS) when I was 13. While nothing in the way of tests was performed, I had several symptoms: facial hair; hair in places I didn't think a girl should have – back, tummy, top of legs, toes; I was overweight; had what I now know was hormonal acne and had had only one period. Other girls around me were getting boobs, bras and discussing periods and buying tampons. I was buying facial hair remover, shavers, hair lightener and acne cream (it never worked). It was a lonely painful existence.

It would take another four years before I had a second period, and even then there followed no pattern: they were sporadic, heavy and painful. In 2013 I was officially diagnosed with PCOS.

I started eating a strict low-carb diet and doing high intensity workouts and from then on my life changed. My periods became regular and lighter, the acne disappeared and weight melted off.

I had been repeatedly told that I would never conceive without medical intervention, but no sooner had we decided to start trying for a baby, I was pregnant!

I still have PCOS, of course, but the symptoms are more controlled as a result of my lifestyle choices.

However, I am still seeking the best cure for hair removal – I don't think that will ever go!

The benefits of a low-carbohydrate, healthy fat approach

Each of the conditions mentioned in the last chapter have two things in common – they are all made worse by high insulin levels, and they can all be improved by reducing insulin levels. There are also other conditions that are associated with obesity but which are not so reversible, including a number of cancers. The risks of colorectal (bowel) cancer, pancreatic cancer and breast cancer are all increased in the presence of increased insulin levels. This is not surprising, as insulin promotes growth, and tumour cells are rapidly growing cells.

The key to reducing insulin levels in the blood is to adopt a healthy diet and increase physical activity. In this context, a healthy diet is one that will actually help reduce insulin levels. The foods that most cause insulin levels to rise are sugars and refined carbohydrates, and there is increasing evidence from a number of studies that high consumption of sugars and refined carbohydrates is associated with increased risk of type 2 diabetes. The strongest association is with the consumption of sugar-sweetened beverages, such as fizzy drinks and fruit juices. However, such associations have also been reported with excess intake of white rice and potatoes, which until recently were regarded as healthier types of carbohydrate. Moreover, while it used to be thought that wholemeal varieties of carbohydrates are less harmful, more recent analysis suggests that the glycaemic index (that is, the rate at which it enters the bloodstream as glucose) of whole wheat bread is even higher than that of French fries or basmati rice, leading many in the medical and dietetic professions to rethink how healthy such 'wholegrain' foods are, especially in a person whose insulin levels are already high.

Much of the evidence for the benefit of a low-carbohydrate diet has come from the treatment of people with obesity and/ or type 2 diabetes, where the emphasis has been to restrict sugars and starchy carbohydrates of all types, regardless of their glycaemic index, as in the end, they are all turned into sugar, and will stimulate the pancreas to release more insulin, thus making the situation worse.

So why does reducing carbohydrates help so much? Just to recap, common to many of the conditions we have discussed, there is insulin resistance.

That means that the insulin produced by the pancreas is ineffective in keeping the level of glucose in the blood stable.

As a result, the pancreas has to produce more insulin in order to have an effect. Although the effect of insulin in stabilising glucose levels is impaired, the insulin that is produced is still very good at its other actions, which are to promote hunger and to store fat. This leads to increased appetite, weight gain and, crucially, storage of fat in the internal organs, particularly the liver and the pancreas. As the level of fat accumulates in the liver, the liver becomes even more resistant to insulin. That means that insulin is less able to control the release of glucose from the liver into the bloodstream, and the level of glucose in the blood rises. In response to this, the pancreas releases even more insulin that leads to yet more appetite stimulation, weight gain and fat in the liver, building up a very vicious circle indeed. In some people, the body is so resistant to insulin that even high levels of insulin are not able to control blood glucose levels, and type 2 diabetes develops; in others, even if they do not develop type 2 diabetes, the high insulin levels contribute to high blood pressure, high cholesterol levels and, in women, to the hormone changes associated with polycystic ovary syndrome.

In using dietary change to manage these conditions, the goal is to consume foods and drinks that will have least effect on blood glucose levels; as a result of less glucose entering the bloodstream from food, the pancreas does not have to produce so much insulin (or in the case of a person with type 1 diabetes, less insulin will need to be injected). This will quite soon lead to less insulin in the bloodstream, which in turn will lead to a reduced sense of hunger and less fat being stored in the liver. Over time, body weight will begin to fall, and the fat in the liver will be used for energy. As the fat content of the liver reduces, the liver will become less resistant to insulin, and as a result, less glucose will be released from the liver stores into the blood. The reduced insulin resistance also means that it is more effective at controlling blood glucose levels, and so the pancreas no longer has to produce so much insulin to get an effect. This then leads to lower levels of insulin in the blood, and correction of the metabolic and hormonal changes that are associated with high insulin levels, so that body weight, blood pressure, cholesterol levels and the hormone changes and symptoms associated with PCOS all begin to improve. Just by changing one's diet, it is possible to break the vicious circle and turn it into a virtuous one, where each improvement leads to still more improvement, with in many cases complete reversal of these health problems.

SO WHAT DOES THIS MEAN IN PRACTICE?

The foods that have the most direct impact on your blood glucose level are sugars and starches. Therefore, in order to eat foods that do not raise blood glucose and insulin levels, it is necessary to reduce your intake of foods containing sugars and starches. This may be the complete opposite of what you have been told previously, as the official UK nutrition advice for the general population and for people with diabetes is to base all meals on starchy carbohydrates. Thankfully however, more and more people are coming to realise that encouraging a person with diabetes, whose body is unable to tolerate carbohydrates, to eat lots of carbohydrates just does not make sense. A low-carbohydrate diet is generally defined as one that contains less than 130 grams of carbohydrate a day. This is about half the average carbohydrate intake of the UK population. I do not advocate firm rules about how much carbohydrate you should eat, but my reading of the evidence is that best and most sustainable results in type 1 and type 2 diabetes are seen in people who eat 50–100 grams of carbohydrate per day. It is likely (but not proven) that the same applies for people with prediabetes, insulin resistance and PCOS.

I therefore generally recommend to aim for less than 100 grams a day, and no more than 25 grams in any one meal. However, I would encourage you to find the level that works well for you and fits in with your own tastes and food preferences. In order to do that, you need to have a good idea about which of the foods you currently eat contain carbohydrate. Full details of this are provided in my previous books, but to recap, starch is found in all grains (including wheat, oats and rice) and products made from them, including cereals, bread and pasta, and in starchy vegetables (mainly root vegetables such as potatoes and parsnips, and legumes such as beans). And sugar is found in fruit and all sweet foods such as biscuits, cakes, desserts, ice cream, sweets, and drinks such as fruit juice and fizzy drinks.

It might be worth having a think about what you currently eat, by engaging in my ten-minute consultation on reducing carbohydrates. It goes something like this. Ask yourself:
• What do you generally eat for breakfast?
• For lunch?
• For your evening meal?
• For snacks?

Typical answers will include cereal and toast for breakfast, perhaps with orange juice, a sandwich or baguette for lunch, maybe with a packet of crisps, and an apple or banana for a snack, or maybe digestive biscuits. Followed by a variety of meals in the evening that usually include potatoes, rice or pasta, which are all carbohydrates of course.

My first suggestion is to avoid cereals at breakfast and to try a breakfast based on eggs (cooked any way, with bacon, tomatoes, mushrooms) or natural yoghurt. I find Greek yoghurt nicer (it has a high protein content and is up to 10 per cent fat!), mixed with a handful of berries, nuts or seeds and perhaps some oats. And, please, no fruit juice.

Lunch could be a homemade soup (avoiding starchy vegetables) or a salad, and if evening meals include some starch, such as bread, rice, potato or pasta, it should occupy just a small corner of the plate if at all, while most of the plate is filled with green vegetables or salad. Better still, try a meal with just protein (such as meat, eggs or fish) and green vegetables. And try and avoid meals based on carbohydrates such as potato or pasta bake, macaroni cheese, pizza or rice dishes.

For snacks, an apple, tangerine, peach, plum or pear are fine (i.e. any small 'round' fruit you can fit in the palm of your hand). Berries are very low in sugar. It is best to avoid eating bananas (unless a small one), pineapple or melon on a regular basis. Try to make up your five-a-day from vegetables rather than fruit. But you could also try a hard-boiled egg, a small piece of cheese or a handful of nuts, which, apart from peanuts and cashews, contain hardly any carbohydrates, but plenty of healthy fats.

With only this modest information to hand, many people have achieved much better control of their diabetes. What is interesting is that by following this advice, people often find they are eating more fresh and natural foods, and less processed food. This means they are also eating less sugar and salt as they are to be found in worrying quantities in just about every type of processed food.

Some people assume that a low-carbohydrate diet has to be high in fat, hence the term 'low-carb, high-fat' or LCHF diet. However studies have shown that this doesn't have to be the case. If you are overweight, reducing starchy carbohydrates and replacing them with generous portions leafy green vegetables will greatly reduce calorie intake and further help weight loss. If you do not need to lose weight, then increasing the portion of protein or of healthy fats, as found in olive oil, avocadoes, nuts, oily fish and dairy products, can make up for the reduced carbohydrates. Thus I prefer to use the term 'low carb, healthy fat' to describe the diet, as by avoiding

processed foods that contain harmful trans fats, and by eating fat found naturally in foods, that is just what it is.

The recipes in this cookbook have all been designed to be consistent with this advice; they provide no more than 25 grams of carbohydrate per serving and they are all low in starches. When trying out a new recipe, you may wish to assess how well your body copes with the meal by checking your blood glucose before and two hours after eating it. If the glucose level remains about the same, you know you can safely eat the meal knowing that it will not push up your glucose level. And that is exactly what you are aiming for!

EMMA: MY LOW-CARB DIET

For me, the benefits of a low-carb diet have been life changing.

First off, I don't starve myself: I eat proper meals and actually eat more now than when I was eating a diet high in carbohydrates, low in fat, and with processed food. My mind is clear and my Hba1c has consistently been around 5.0 per cent.

By eating this way, I've also managed to banish the following persistent health issues:

- Headaches. Something I used to suffer from on a daily basis.

- Irregular periods. My periods are now much more frequent. I have also managed to get pregnant and become a mum naturally, something I was told would not be possible as a type 1 diabetic with PCOS.

- Acne. I used to be prone to erratic and painful acne around my jaw, chin, back and chest.

- Bloating. I used to frequently feel bloated and 'heavy' and would regularly rush home from work to throw on the baggiest clothes I could find to liberate my tummy.

And the following things have dramatically improved:

- Energy.

- Lack of cravings. I no longer have any of my old cravings for chocolate or Diet Coke. If I crave anything now, I make sure that I make it from scratch myself using fresh ingredients.

- Libido.

- Skin. My skin is clear, I don't have to hide behind layers of make-up and I don't get breakouts.

- Hair. It's shinier, healthier, thicker, longer and less brittle.

- Feeling fuller and more satisfied after meals.

- My mind is clearer and I feel more positive.

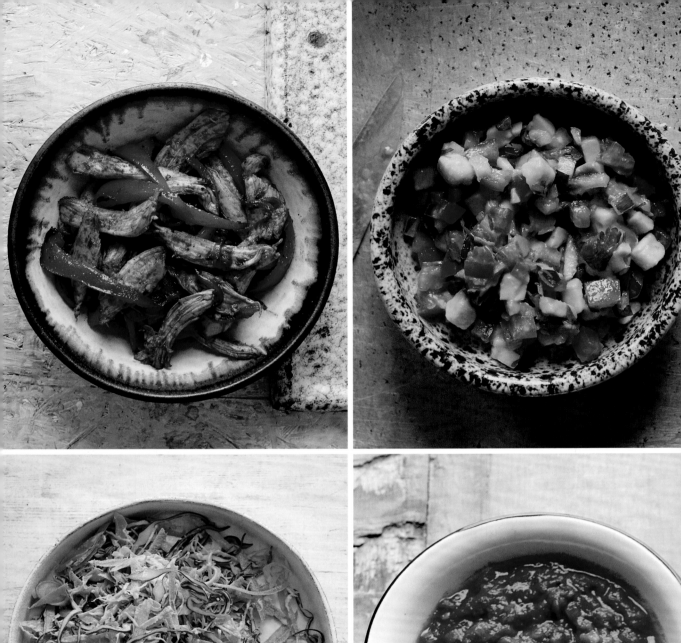
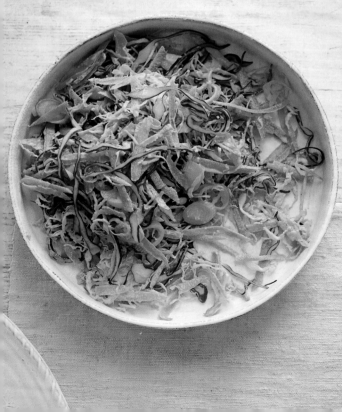
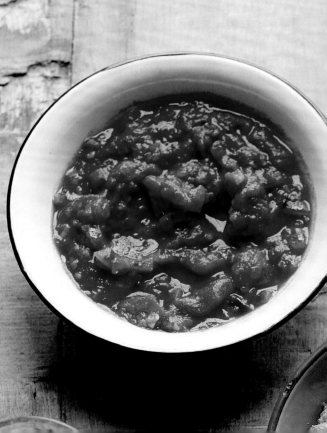

Kitchen Cupboard Essentials

———●○●———

With a low-carb diet, you can soon end up thinking 'What *can* I eat?' and, as you start to focus on eating well, it is hard to resist the endless temptations of high-calorific, sugar-laden food. Even with the best of intentions it is all too easy to end up with a trolley full of biscuits and cakes. I've been there, trust me! Source the best food you can afford – especially eggs, meat and fish. Always read ingredients labels and check for any hidden additives. Try to shop alone, with a list, a full tummy and a bottle of water. These kitchen cupboard essentials are foods I use on a regular basis and with a huge variety of healthy ingredients out there, I hope you will enjoy adding them to *your* kitchen cupboard.

NUTS AND SEEDS

Nuts and seeds are low in carbs and full of healthy fats, vitamins and minerals. However, stick to a handful of nuts or seeds and always be mindful of portion size. Avoid nuts roasted with added salt, and make sure nut and seed butters are just made of nuts or seeds, with no added oils or salts/sugars. You can also make your own (see page 71).

- almonds
- cashew nuts
- chia seeds
- hazelnuts
- macadamia nuts
- pumpkin seeds
- sunflower seeds
- walnuts

NUT AND SEED BUTTERS

- almond nut butter
- cashew nut butter
- hazelnut butter
- pumpkin seed butter
- tahini (sesame)

FATS FOR COOKING

Contrary to popular belief, healthy fats are extremely good for you and despite fat having more calories per gram than protein or carbohydrates, diets high in healthy fats are not going to make you fat! The fats you should eliminate from your diet are industrial vegetable oils such as sunflower oil, corn oil, canola oil, peanut oil, sesame oil, low-fat spreads and margarine. Healthy fats include:

- avocado oil
- coconut oil
- full-fat butter/ghee
- macadamia nut oil
- olive oil

COCONUT MILK

Buy high-quality coconut milk, free from added preservatives and stabilisers. You are more likely to find organic brands that are BPA and/or guar gum-free in health-food stores.

FLOUR

Nut or seed flours (such as ground almonds, sesame flour and coconut flour) are a brilliant substitute for high-carb wheat flours. They are gluten and grain free and although they won't have the same springiness that you get in gluten-based baked goods, they contain much fewer carbs and as such will help you maintain a much more stable blood sugar level. Be wary of 'free-from' flours which are still high in carbs.

EGGS

Eggs are one of the most nutritious, affordable, easy-to-cook, protein-packed foods. Low in carbs, they don't inflate blood sugars and they contain all the essential amino acids and promote a feeling of fullness. Buy free range and organic if possible.

SPICES

Spices can transform a dish and have incredible health-boosting properties, with many being high in antioxidants and vitamins. Some also have anti-inflammatory benefits. I always have these and flaky sea salt to hand:

- black pepper
- cardamom
- cayenne
- cinnamon
- cloves
- chilli
- cumin
- fennel seeds
- ginger
- garam masala
- nutmeg
- paprika
- turmeric
- vanilla

HERBS

Fresh or dried, herbs add flavour to food and are full of nutritional goodness. My favourites include:

- basil
- bay leaves
- coriander
- dill
- mint
- oregano
- parsley
- rosemary
- sage
- tarragon
- thyme

MEAT AND FISH

Buy the best meat and fish you can afford. It's better for you (not pumped with additives, sugars and water), more ethical and reduces your carbon footprint. Buy from your local butcher, fishmonger or farmers' market when possible.

FRUIT AND VEGETABLES

Most fruits are very high in sugar and should be enjoyed in moderation. However, berries are lower in sugar and high in antioxidants and a daily handful makes a healthy snack. Avoid dried fruits because they have a concentrated and high sugar content. Enjoy vegetables in abundance, especially green and leafy ones. Be wary of root vegetables as they have a higher carb content and will require strict portion control. Here are some of my favourite fruit and vegetables:

FRUIT

- apples (great for sauces, smoothies or cakes)
- avocado (blood-sugar friendly, full of good fats and filling)
- bananas (useful in baking but very high in carbs)
- berries (blueberry, blackberry, strawberry)
- cherries
- coconut
- tomatoes
- olives (carb friendly and a good snack)
- watermelon

VEGETABLES

- artichokes
- asparagus
- aubergine
- bell peppers
- beetroot
- bok choi
- butternut squash
- Brussels sprouts
- broccoli
- cabbage
- carrots
- celery
- cauliflower
- cucumber
- courgette
- garlic
- kale
- leeks
- lettuce
- mushrooms
- onions
- parsnips
- radish
- rocket
- seaweed
- spinach
- sweet potatoes
- Swiss chard
- watercress

DAIRY

Avoid low-fat dairy and dairy products with added sugar or sweeteners. Buy natural, full-fat plain yoghurt. Full-fat dairy products are a very good source of prebiotics, protein and calcium.

MILK ALTERNATIVES

If you are avoiding dairy you can make your own nut milk alternatives (almonds or cashews – pages 64–67) or buy them, or coconut milk, from supermarkets; go for unsweetened versions, not low-fat or sweetened ones.

CHOCOLATE

Cacao is cocoa in its rawest form, and it's great for giving smoothies, desserts and cakes a rich chocolate flavour. If you can't find it, use unsweetened cocoa powder. There's no point living life without the odd treat. I love 85 per cent cocoa chocolate: it has limited impact on sugar levels and the higher the percentage of cocoa solids, the lower the sugar content.

DRINKS

Water is the best thing you can drink. If you can't give up coffee or tea, or other cafffeinated drinks, avoid adding sugar and sweeteners. Herbal teas are a flavourful, healthier alternative to sugary soft drinks. To make a herbal iced tea:

- Add a herbal teabag to a glass. Pour 2.5cm of boiling water over it. Leave to infuse for 10 minutes. Add ice (crushed or cubed) and cover with cold water.

Or, try flavoured water:

- Blitz strawberries and blueberries in a blender, pour into a glass, add crushed ice and top up with still or sparkling water.

Drinks can conceal so many added sugars. Be aware that alcoholic drinks like cocktails can contain added sugar, syrups, sugary liqueurs and fruit juice. If I am having alcohol I opt for a vodka soda with a squeeze of lime. The only time I use fruit juice is to treat a low blood sugar: it's my medicine and can quite literally save my life.

NUTRITIONAL INFORMATION

The nutritional information listed with each recipe does not include the nutritional content of garnishes or any optional accompaniments, and is for one serving per person in accordance with strict portion control. It is an estimate only and may vary depending on the brand of ingredients you use, and due to natural biological variations in the composition of natural foods.

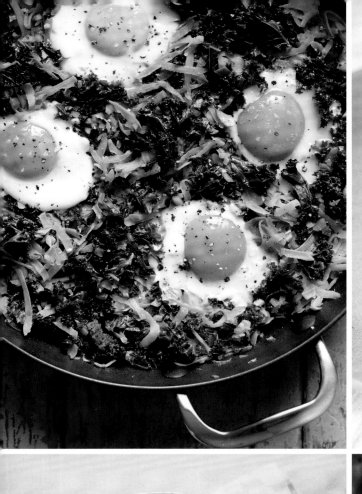

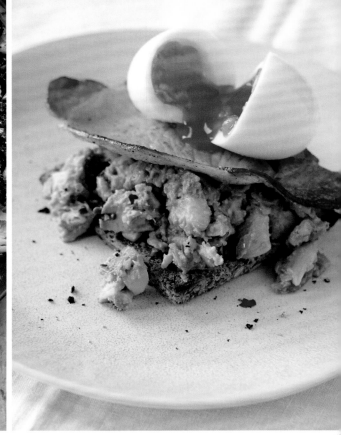

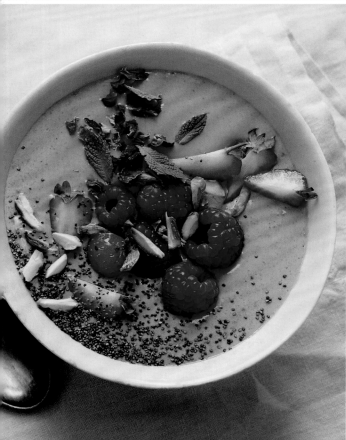

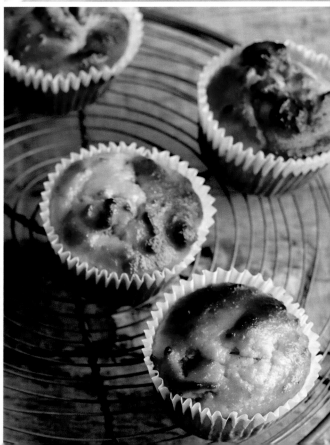

Breakfasts

How to MAKE AN OMELETTE

This may sound obvious, but over the years I have had omelettes made in various ways, many of which have been far too complicated. If you want to make them well, try this simple method for the perfect omelette.

Eggs are brilliant for breakfast, lunch, dinner or a snack: there really isn't a bad time to eat them. They are loaded with protein, vitamins, minerals and healthy fats and are very low in carbs, too, which means that they will keep you feeling fuller for longer.

 1   2 MINS   7 MINS

3 medium eggs
knob of butter
sea salt and cracked black
 pepper

1. Crack the eggs into a bowl and whisk until smooth, then season with salt and pepper.

2. Place a non-stick frying pan over medium heat and add the butter.

3. Once the butter starts to sizzle, pour in the beaten egg.

4. Using a spatula, carefully drag the outer edges of the omelette, where it is starting to stick, into the middle of the pan. Fill any gaps in the egg mix by tilting the pan from side to side. Do this a couple of times until the mixture is starting to set.

5. Cook for 2–3 minutes, then carefully fold the omelette in half using the spatula and slide it onto a plate.

SOME FILLING TIPS:
If you are adding fillings, cook the ingredients first then add the egg mixture. If you are adding cheese, scatter it over the centre of the cooked omelette so it can melt before you fold it over.

MY TOP OMELETTE-MAKING TIPS:
o Buy the best-quality eggs you can afford.
o Use unsalted full-fat butter to fry them, rather than margarine or any other oils.
o Beat the eggs well in a bowl or jug before pouring them into the pan. Make sure there are no flecks of white and the mixture is completely combined.
o Use a non-stick frying pan and make sure that the butter is fully melted before you pour in the eggs.
o Do not cook an omelette over high heat. Use a medium heat and cook it slowly so that the egg doesn't burn.

NUTRITIONAL INFORMATION

Calories	Carbs
272	2g
Total Fat	**Protein**
21g	19g

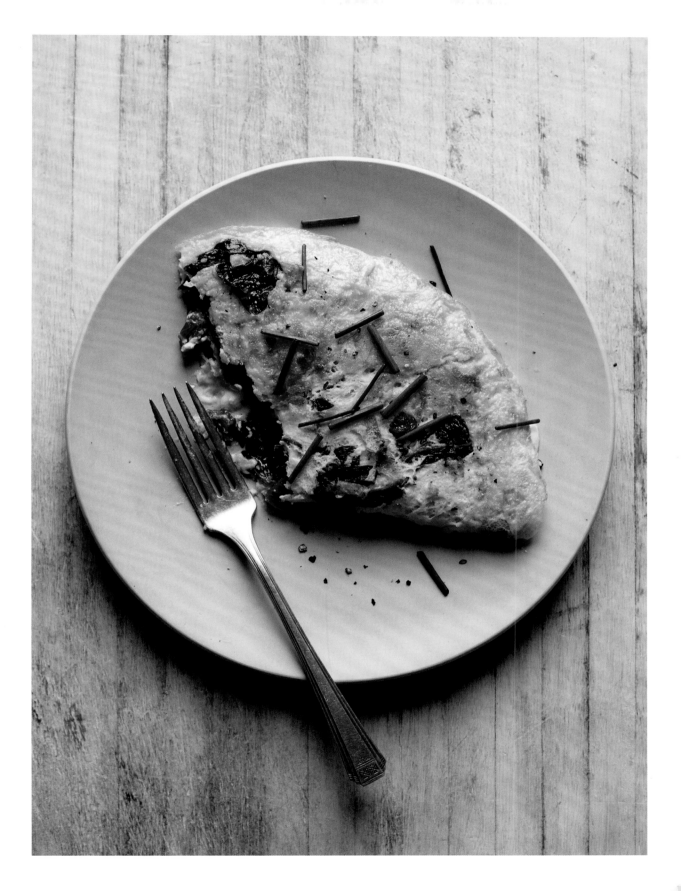

blueberry and cinnamon omelette

This delicious protein-packed breakfast, a satisfying and speedy omelette with the delicious natural sweetness of blueberries and cinnamon, is perfect for those seeking a sweeter dish without all the carbs you find in a cereal-based breakfast.

 1   **2 MINS**   **7 MINS**

3 eggs
1 tsp ground cinnamon
1 tsp coconut oil
a handful of blueberries
a few pumpkin seeds, to serve (optional)

1. Crack the eggs into a bowl, add the cinnamon and whisk until smooth.

2. Place a non-stick frying pan over medium heat, and add the coconut oil. Once melted, put half the blueberries into the frying pan and cook for about 30 seconds until softened.

3. Pour in the egg mixture and, using a spatula, carefully drag the outer edges of the omelette, where it is starting to stick, into the middle of the pan.

4. Fill any gaps in the egg mix by tilting the pan from side to side. Do this a couple of times until the mixture is starting to set.

5. Scatter the remaining blueberries over the omelette and turn the heat down to low, then cook for 2–3 minutes before carefully folding the omelette in half using the spatula and sliding it onto a plate.

6. Serve immediately with a sprinkling of pumpkin seeds, if using.

ALTERNATIVE SWEET OPTIONS, FOLLOWING THE SAME METHOD:

o A handful of raspberries (about 6 whole ones) with a pinch of vanilla seeds added to the egg mixture before adding fruit as above.

o 40g thinly sliced banana and ½ teaspoon ground cinnamon added to the egg mixture before adding fruit as above.

o A handful of blackberries (about 5 whole ones) and ½ apple, grated and added to the egg mixture before adding fruit as above.

o 2 strawberries and a handful of blueberries served with 1 tablespoon full-fat Greek yoghurt.

NUTRITIONAL INFORMATION

Calories	Carbs
311	12g
Total Fat	Protein
23g	20g

spinach, sun-dried tomato and goat's cheese omelette

Don't skip breakfast – try this! With a few simple ingredients, you can have this deliciously satisfying, low-carb and nutritious meal on the table in under ten minutes. Or make it the night before, roll it up, cut it in half and eat it on the go! It could also be enjoyed as a lunch or a light supper.

 1   2 MINS   7 MINS

3 eggs

knob of butter

a handful of spinach leaves

3 whole sun-dried tomatoes from a jar, drained and chopped into small pieces

2 slices (40g) of your favourite goat's cheese, crumbled

sea salt and cracked black pepper

a few chives, chopped, to garnish

1. Crack the eggs into a bowl and season with salt and pepper.

2. Melt the butter in a non-stick frying pan over medium heat. Once the butter starts to sizzle, add the spinach and chopped sun-dried tomatoes. Fry for 40–60 seconds until the spinach has softened a little, then pour in the egg mixture and, using a spatula, carefully drag the outer edges of the omelette, where it is starting to stick, into the middle of the pan.

3. Fill any gaps in the egg mix by tilting the pan from side to side. Do this a couple of times until the mixture is starting to set.

4. Scatter the crumbled goat's cheese over the omelette, then cook for 2–3 minutes before carefully folding the omelette in half using the spatula and sliding it onto a plate.

5. Serve immediately with a sprinkling of chives.

ALTERNATIVE SAVOURY OPTIONS, FOLLOWING THE SAME METHOD:

○ Sliced chorizo (40g) and ¼ thinly sliced red onion.

○ ½ sliced avocado and 3 sliced cherry tomatoes, with grated Cheddar cheese (45g). Add avocado before folding omelette.

○ Sliced tomato (90g), grated Cheddar cheese (50g) and 5 finely chopped basil leaves. Cook the tomato before adding the egg and remaining ingredients.

○ 3 sliced mushrooms, sliced red pepper (40g) and crumbled feta (40g). Cook mushrooms and pepper then add egg and feta.

○ Sliced butcher's unsmoked ham, sliced and halved, ½ small aubergine, sliced widthways and cut in half, and 3 sun-dried tomatoes. You will need to cook the aubergine for a little longer until soft.

NUTRITIONAL INFORMATION

Calories	Carbs
430	8g
Total Fat	**Protein**
32g	29g

one-pan bacon, eggs and asparagus

This is such a simple breakfast but the flavour combinations are a match made in breakfast heaven. The only seasoning I would use is lots of cracked black pepper; with the bacon it's salty enough. As a one-pan dish, it's quick to make and involves little washing up.

If you have one, use a non-stick frying pan to dry-fry this breakfast without added fat; if not, use a knob of butter. For a vegetarian breakfast, substitute some thickly sliced mushrooms for the bacon – if you omit the bacon, add a little sea salt and maybe some coriander or parsley to pep up the dish.

 4　 **5 MINS**　 **10–12 MINS**

8 medium asparagus spears (about 128g), woody ends snapped off

4 dry-cured, thick-cut back bacon rashers

4 large eggs

cracked black pepper

1. Dry-fry the asparagus in a non-stick pan for 1–2 minutes, then add about 2 tablespoons of water to help them soften a little but so they still retain a slight crunch.

2. Once the water has evaporated, add the bacon rashers and cook for 1 minute on each side.

3. Crack the eggs into the pan, one at a time, keeping the heat at medium. Cooking the eggs will take a few minutes, but it will be worth the wait.

4. Transfer to a serving plate, add plenty of cracked black pepper and enjoy with a big pot of steaming tea. You could also serve this on a slice of Super seed bread (see page 198).

NOTE: The better quality the bacon, the less water it will contain, and therefore the more it will retain its shape and size.

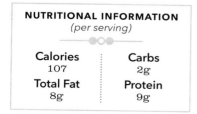

NUTRITIONAL INFORMATION
(per serving)

Calories	Carbs
107	2g
Total Fat	**Protein**
8g	9g

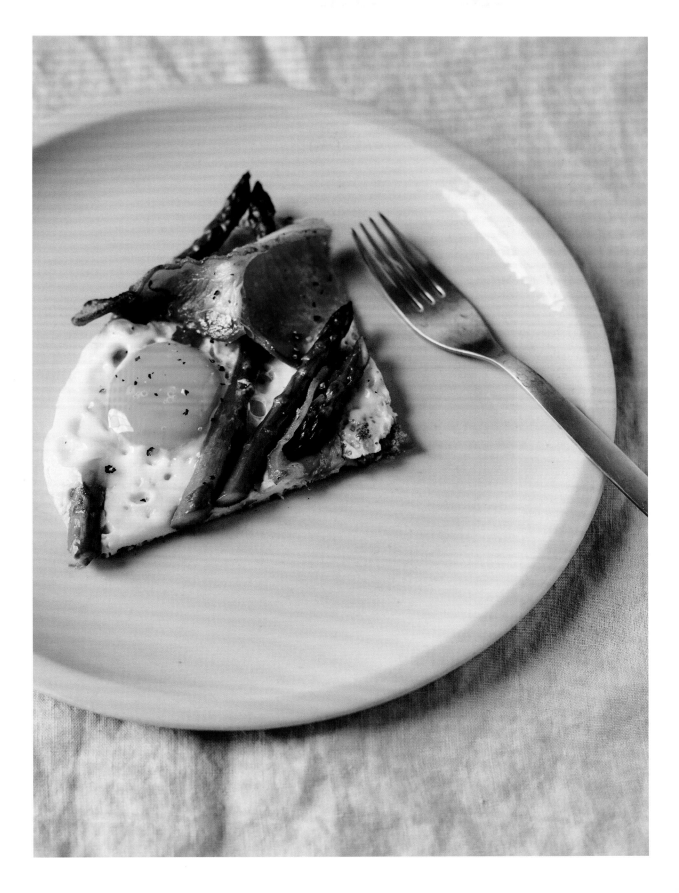

sweet potato and kale rosti with baked eggs

I created this a few years ago and it has since become one of the most popular recipes on my blog; it's also one of my favourites to make on a Saturday morning for guests. It's bright, vibrant and packed with flavour and texture, as well as protein and all the vital vitamins and nutrients. Quick, simple and only one pan needed – perfect for slicing and sharing.

 4   10 MINS   12–15 MINS

230g sweet potato, peeled

1 tsp coconut oil or butter

240g red onion, finely chopped

3 garlic cloves, finely chopped

½ tsp sea salt

2 large handfuls of kale, chopped

4 large eggs

juice of ½ lime

cracked black pepper

a small handful of coriander leaves, chopped, to garnish

dried chilli flakes, to taste (optional)

1. Using a food processor fitted with the 'grating' attachment, coarsely grate the sweet potato – you can use a box grater instead, but you will need plenty of elbow grease!

2. Melt the coconut oil or butter in a non-stick frying pan over medium-high heat. Add the grated sweet potato and fry for 2–3 minutes until it softens. Add the red onion and garlic and fry for a further 3–4 minutes until the onion softens and is translucent.

3. Add the salt and place the kale on top of the vegetables, letting the leaves steam a little before mixing them in. You will be amazed at how much the volume of kale reduces and how quickly!

4. Firmly press the mix down and reduce the heat to medium, to avoid the bottom burning.

5. Crack the eggs on top and leave to cook through for 6–7 minutes.

6. You can finish the dish off under the grill if you like a crisp top – I don't usually do this, however, as I prefer my yolks runny.

7. Once everything is cooked through, drizzle the lime juice over the dish, scatter over the chopped coriander to garnish and add some cracked black pepper and dried chilli to taste, if you like.

8. Serve immediately or allow to cool, then slice up and enjoy when ready.

NUTRITIONAL INFORMATION
(per serving)

Calories	Carbs
181	23g
Total Fat	**Protein**
7g	9g

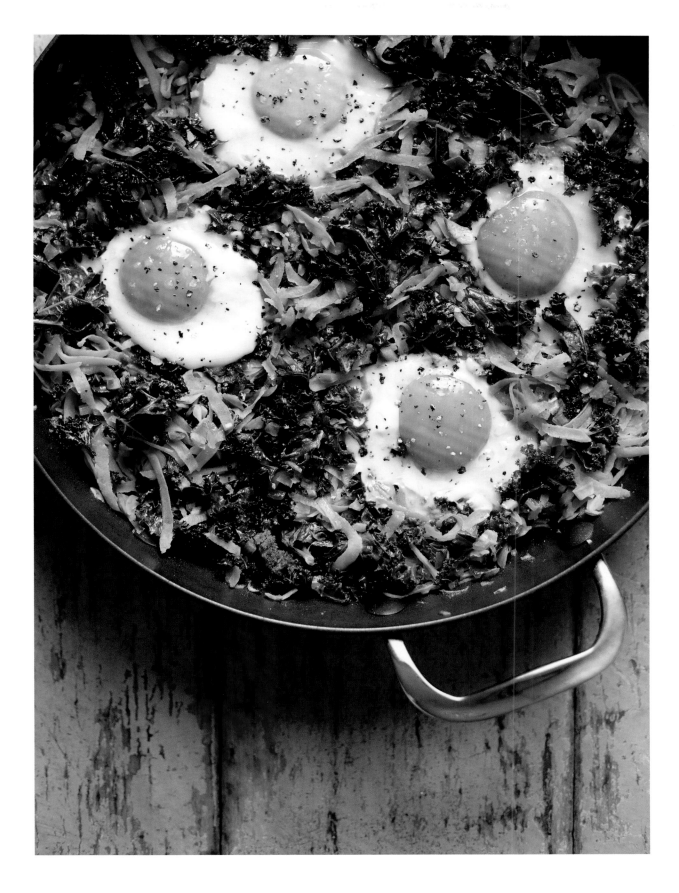

crushed avocado toast
with soft-boiled egg and bacon

A delicious twist on a classic brunch favourite. This simple recipe is perfect when you need a quick and nutritious breakfast. Crisp bacon, cool whipped-up avocado, a perfectly cooked soft-boiled egg with a golden yolk and warm, buttery toast. A sure-fire way to get people out of bed!

Double the ingredients if you are making the dish for two and quadruple them for four.

 1   **10 MINS**   **10–12 MINS**

1 large egg

1 small ripe avocado, halved, de-stoned and peeled

a pinch of dried chilli flakes

1 rasher of unsmoked back bacon

1 slice of Super seed bread (see page 198)

knob of butter, for spreading

sea salt and cracked black pepper

1. Bring 500ml of water to the boil in a small pan over high heat.

2. Carefully lower the egg into the boiling water, then boil for exactly 6 minutes, making sure the egg is completely submerged in the water at all times.

3. Remove the egg from the pan and immediately place it under cold running water for 2–3 minutes to ensure the egg cools and stops cooking, then set aside.

4. Scoop the avocado flesh into a bowl, add the dried chilli flakes and season with salt and pepper. Take a fork and crush the avocado until it has broken up and is well combined with the other ingredients.

5. Heat a non-stick frying pan or griddle pan over medium heat and dry-fry the bacon for 2–3 minutes on each side until cooked through.

6. Toast the Super seed bread in a toaster or under the grill.

7. Slather the toast with butter, then top with the crushed avocado mixture and pop the bacon rasher on top.

8. Carefully peel the boiled egg and add it to the stack, then cut it in half and allow the soft yolk to spill over the bacon, avocado and toast.

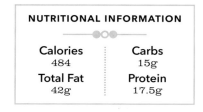

NUTRITIONAL INFORMATION

Calories	Carbs
484	15g
Total Fat	**Protein**
42g	17.5g

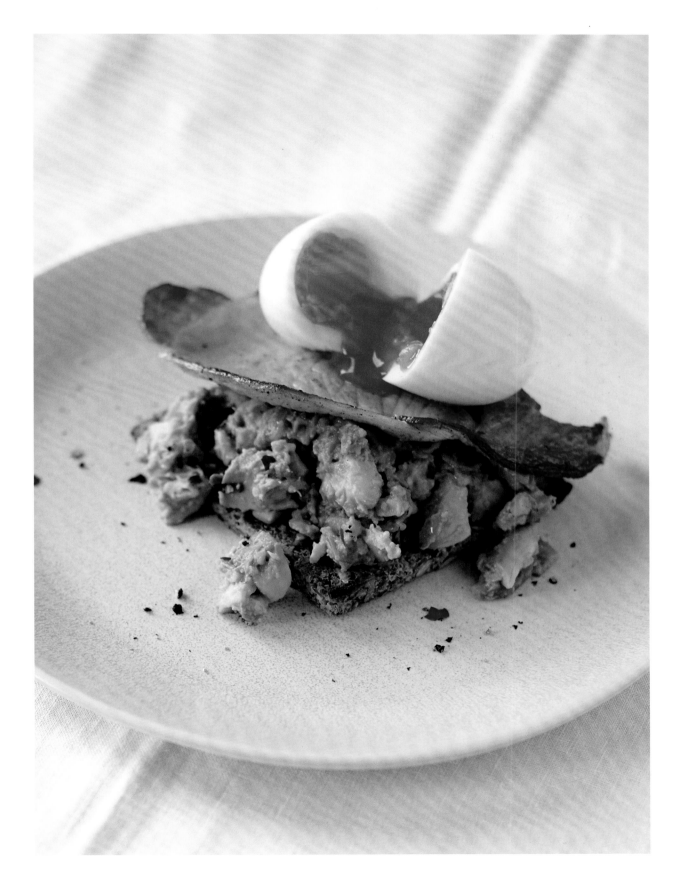

baked eggs in avocado with roasted fennel and tomatoes

Here's a simple and nutritious breakfast for the weekend, when you have time to cook, eat and relax. This is a breakfast to really sit and savour.

Eggs and avocado work beautifully together at any time, but when baked together they are really at their best. Full of healthy fats and low in carbs, this dish is ideal for sharing. The addition of the roasted fennel and tomatoes brings extra flavour and makes this perfect for a weekend brunch.

 4   **10 MINS**   **20–25 MINS**

For the baked avocados

- 2 large avocados (about 440g), halved and de-stoned
- 4 eggs

For the roasted fennel and tomatoes

- 130g cherry tomatoes
- 2 fennel bulbs (about 180g), stalks removed, bulbs thinly sliced from top to bottom
- 1 tbsp olive oil, plus extra for greasing
- sea salt and cracked black pepper

1. Preheat the oven to 200°C/400°F/gas mark 6 and lightly grease 2 baking trays.

2. Using a spoon, scoop out a little extra flesh from the avocado halves where the stone was to create a decent well for the egg – it needs to be deep enough to accommodate the egg and all the white, without spilling. Place the avocado halves on one of the baking trays.

3. Gently crack an egg into the well of each avocado, being careful not to split the yolk.

4. Place in the oven and bake for 20–25 minutes until the egg whites and yolks have set.

5. Spread the cherry tomatoes and fennel slices onto the other greased baking tray. Drizzle with the olive oil and season with salt and pepper, and put the tray into the oven to cook while the avocado cooks. Bake for about 12 minutes, remove the tray and quickly turn the fennel slices, then bake for a further 10 minutes until the tomatoes are caramelising and the fennel is soft with browned edges.

6. Remove from the oven and serve the baked avocados immediately with the roasted fennel and tomatoes.

NUTRITIONAL INFORMATION
(per serving)

Calories	Carbs
292	13g
Total Fat	**Protein**
25g	10g

baked breakfast mushrooms

This is a really straightforward breakfast that looks good and tastes great. With only three key ingredients, some seasoning and a little garnish, it's a low-carb showstopper that's meaty, filling, quick to make and full of protein. Always opt for the best bacon and eggs you can afford – organic and free range when possible.

 4   **5 MINS**   **20 MINS**

1 tbsp olive oil, plus extra for greasing

4 large flat mushrooms, stalks removed

2 rashers of unsmoked back bacon, cut into strips widthways

4 large eggs

1 tsp cracked black pepper

coriander leaves, to garnish (optional)

1. Preheat the oven to 200°C /400°F/gas mark 6 and lightly grease a baking tray.

2. Place the mushrooms on the baking tray, stalk-side up, and drizzle each with the olive oil.

3. Pop 3–4 strips of bacon into the middle of each mushroom, then one by one carefully crack the eggs and drop one into the centre of each mushroom (being careful not to split the yolk!).

4. Place the remaining strips of bacon on top of the egg before seasoning with the pepper and placing in the oven for 20 minutes until baked and firm.

5. Serve straightaway, garnished with some coriander if you like, or allow to cool then place in a sealed container to chill and eat within 2 days.

NUTRITIONAL INFORMATION
(per serving)

Calories	Carbs
143	5g
Total Fat	**Protein**
10g	11g

sweet potato, green cabbage and red onion hash with fried peppered eggs

This is a great brunch dish for two hungry people, or for four with a side of toast (see page 198) and some roasted fennel and tomatoes (see page 44). It is an easy one-pan dish packed full of delicious flavours. The fried peppered eggs with deep runny yolks complete this perfectly. It is blood sugar-friendly food for the whole family to enjoy.

 4   10 MINS   11–17 MINS

200g sweet potato, peeled and grated

1 tbsp olive oil

½ medium red onion (about 90g), thinly sliced

190g white cabbage, thinly sliced

5 large eggs (1 for the hash, plus 1 fried egg each, so if serving fewer people, reduce numbers accordingly)

sea salt and cracked black pepper

1. Put the peeled and grated sweet potato into a clean tea towel, nut milk bag or muslin square and squeeze out any water.

2. Pour the olive oil into a non-stick frying pan over medium-high heat. Fry the onion and sweet potato for about 3 minutes until soft, then add the cabbage and fry for 3–4 minutes until it begins to wilt.

3. Reduce the heat to low. Add 1 of the eggs and roughly scrape it up in the pan to combine it with the vegetable mixture, then spread the hash evenly over the bottom of the pan.

4. Crack in the remaining eggs on top of the hash, two on each, and add a generous amount of pepper.

5. Fry over low heat for 5–10 minutes until the whites have cooked and the yolks are firm but still runny.

6. Season well with salt and serve straightaway.

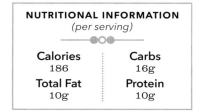

NUTRITIONAL INFORMATION
(per serving)

Calories	Carbs
186	16g
Total Fat	**Protein**
10g	10g

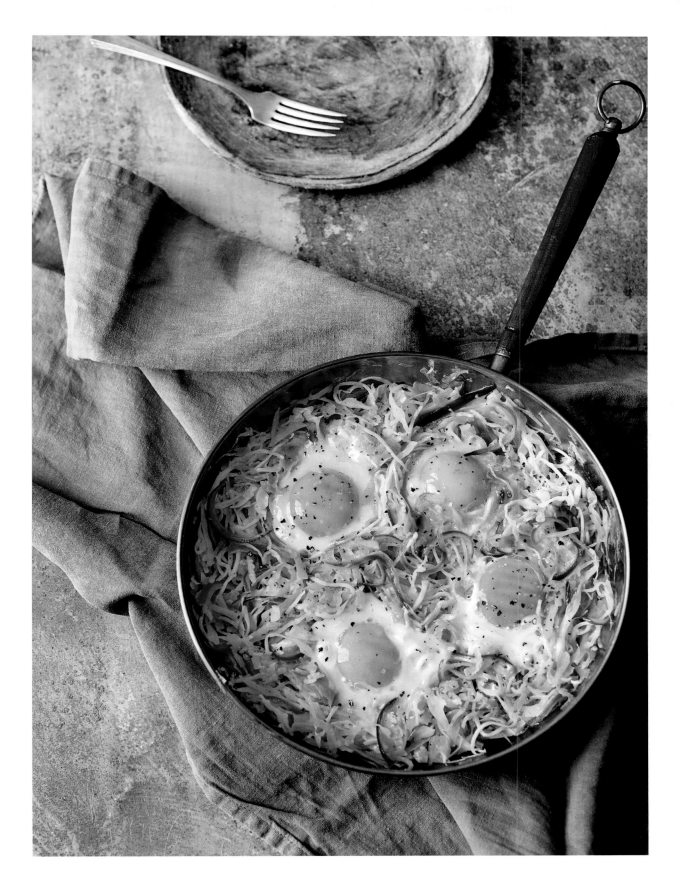

green eggs with avocado and tomato salsa

These green eggs are so simple to make and perfect to share among four people for a big breakfast feast. A filling yet very low-carb dish, it's packed with protein and healthy fats. I like to serve it with my grain-free bread (see page 198), toasting the bread then topping it with the eggs and salsa, which is a delicious accompaniment and is best made just before serving. This is a great way to start your day and keep your blood sugars stable.

 4   **10 MINS**   **4–6 MINS**

For the green eggs

5 large eggs

knob of butter

6 spring onions (about 90g), thinly sliced

2 handfuls of spinach, chopped

6 basil leaves, chopped

sea salt and black pepper

Super seed bread (see page 198), to serve

For the avocado and tomato salsa

5 ripe tomatoes (about 500g), finely chopped

½ red onion (about 110g), finely diced

1 large ripe avocado, halved, de-stoned, peeled and cubed

3 tbsp olive oil

grated zest and juice of 1 lime

a handful of coriander, finely chopped

1. First, prepare the salsa. Put the chopped tomatoes, onion and avocado in a serving bowl. Drizzle over the olive oil and mix well, then add the lime zest and juice to taste. Season with salt and scatter over the chopped coriander.

2. Now, prepare the eggs. Beat the eggs together in a bowl until fully combined, then season to taste.

3. Melt the butter in a frying pan (preferably non-stick) over medium heat, then add the spring onions and fry for 2–3 minutes until softened. Add the spinach and basil and fry for a minute to allow the leaves to soften slightly.

4. Add the egg mix and slowly, using a spatula, start scraping the egg around the frying pan as it cooks. Reduce the heat to low and continue to scrape the egg around the pan for about 2–3 minutes until cooked but still creamy or at the desired consistency.

5. Serve straightaway on toasted seed bread with a generous twist of cracked black pepper and the avocado and tomato salsa.

NUTRITIONAL INFORMATION *(per serving)*					
green eggs		*seed bread*		*avocado salsa*	
Calories	Carbs	Calories	Carbs	Calories	Carbs
128	3g	171	6g	204	12g
Total Fat	Protein	Total Fat	Protein	Total Fat	Protein
10g	9g	15g	8g	18g	3g

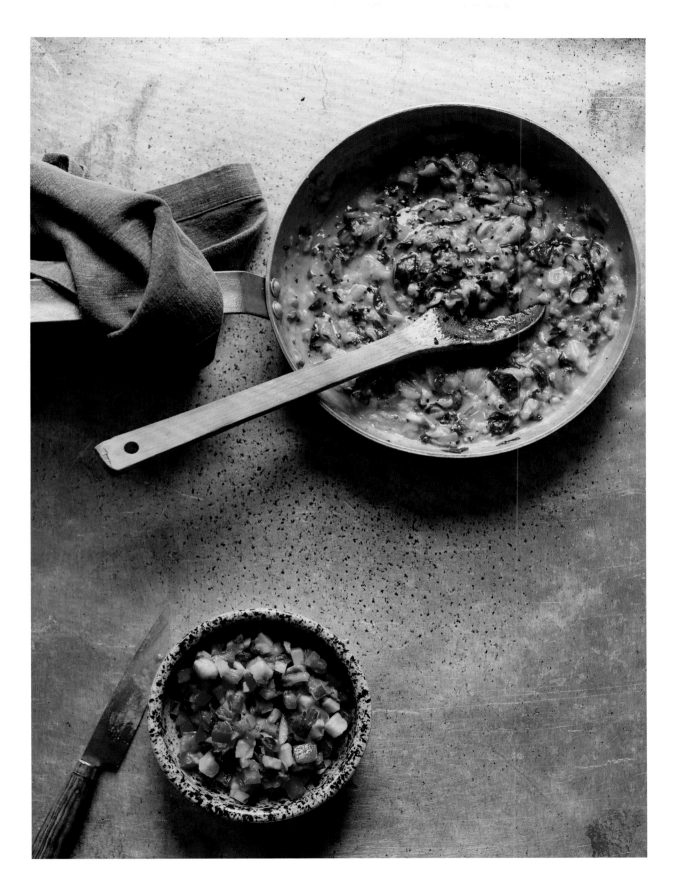

zesty lime, courgette and spring onion fritters

This simple savoury breakfast dish really couldn't be any more perfect and is one that the whole family will love. The word fritter suggests deep-fried and greasy food, but these are light and wonderfully zesty.

Great served hot or cold, these fritters can be enjoyed on the go or at the kitchen table. You can make them whatever size works best for you; I like to make them palm size so that they are easy to hold.

My favourite way to serve them is as a weekend brunch alongside some homemade guacamole and scrambled eggs.

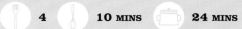 4   10 MINS   24 MINS

250g courgette, coarsely grated

20g spring onion, finely chopped

juice of ½ lime

30g ground almonds or almond flour

2 large eggs, beaten

3 tsp coconut oil

sea salt and cracked black pepper

2 limes, cut into wedges, to serve

1. It's important to drain as much water from the courgette as possible otherwise your fritters may be soggy: place the grated courgette in a nut milk bag or muslin and carefully squeeze out any excess moisture.

2. Put the drained grated courgette, spring onion, lime juice and ground almonds or almond flour in a mixing bowl and season well with salt and pepper. Gradually add the beaten eggs and mix thoroughly until you have a thick, lumpy batter.

3. Melt the coconut oil in a frying pan over high heat, then place 1 heaped tablespoon of batter in the pan and spread it out a little so that it is about 2cm thick.

4. Allow the underside to cook for 2–3 minutes until golden and easy to lift with a spatula, then carefully turn over the fritter and cook the other side for 2–3 minutes until golden brown. Repeat until you have used all the batter.

5. Serve the fritters straight from the pan with wedges of lime or allow to cool and enjoy later.

NUTRITIONAL INFORMATION
(per serving of 2 fritters)

Calories	Carbs
124	4g
Total Fat	**Protein**
11g	6g

sweet potato, leek and lime fritters

The great thing about these fritters is that they are just as good eaten straight from the oven or cold from the fridge (where they can be kept in a sealed container for up to 5 days). They are really filling and have the same satisfying bite that we all seem to crave at any time of day!

You can make them thick or thin; I usually make them about 2cm thick and have one or two at a time. If I am at home and have time I'll slice up some avocado and cook some mushrooms in butter to accompany them. Or I'll pop a couple in a Tupperware and eat them on the go.

 4   **10** MINS   **13–15** MINS

350g sweet potato, peeled and grated

150g leek, thinly sliced

2 tsp grated lime zest

2 tbsp coconut flour

1–2 tbsp coconut oil, plus extra for greasing

3 large eggs, beaten

sea salt and cracked black pepper

juice of 2 limes

1. Preheat the oven to 200°C/400°F/gas mark 6 and grease a baking sheet.

2. Place the grated sweet potato in a large bowl with the leek, lime zest and coconut flour. Season to taste, stir the mixture together, then slowly add the beaten eggs and mix to form a batter.

3. Melt 1 tablespoon of the coconut oil in a deep-sided frying pan over high heat. Spoon 1 tablespoon of the mixture into the pan and spread to about 2cm thick.

4. Add in up to 4 fritters at a time, with a little more coconut oil, if needed, and cook for 2–3 minutes to allow the underside to turn golden brown before flipping carefully and cooking the other side for another 2 minutes. Both sides should be nicely browned. Set aside and continue until you have used all the batter.

5. Place all the fritters on the greased baking sheet and pop in the oven to cook for 5 minutes to ensure they are cooked through.

6. Once cooked, squeeze a generous amount of lime juice over them and serve straightaway or allow to cool and serve later.

NOTE: If your mixture is too dry, add another egg, but 3 large eggs should be plenty.

NUTRITIONAL INFORMATION
(per serving of 2 fritters)

Calories	Carbs
100	13g
Total Fat	**Protein**
4g	4g

sausage, red onion, sun-dried tomato and spinach frittata

Frittatas are great as you can jam as much goodness into them as you want; the eggs provide all the protein you need for the day, and it's low carb, too. It probably looks a lot more sophisticated than it is, but this is just a chuck-it-all-into-the-pan kind of dish.

Delicious hot or cold, cut it into pizza-like slices, pop in a Tupperware, take to work, eat on the bus or have it at a picnic. It's also great served with a little avocado for breakfast or a side salad for lunch.

 4   **10 MINS**   **24–26 MINS**

2 tbsp olive oil

4 sausages (100 per cent organic meat if possible)

150g red onions, diced

50g sun-dried tomatoes from a jar, drained and roughly chopped

100g spinach leaves

¼ tsp dried oregano

¼ tsp dried basil

¼ tsp dried thyme

¼ tsp dried rosemary

¼ tsp dried sage

8 large eggs, beaten

sea salt and cracked black pepper

1 tsp grated lemon zest, to serve

about 20g Parmesan, grated, to serve

1. Preheat the grill to high.

2. Heat 1 tablespoon of the olive oil in a large, non-stick, ovenproof frying pan. Add the sausages and fry over medium heat for 8–10 minutes, turning them occasionally until they are evenly browned.

3. Remove the sausages from the pan, chop them into bite-sized chunks and leave to cool a little.

4. While the sausages are cooling, wipe the pan and pour in the remaining olive oil, then add the red onion and cook over medium heat for about 3 minutes until soft. Add the sun-dried tomatoes and half the spinach and wait for the leaves to wilt a little – about 1 minute – before returning the sausages to the pan. Add all the herbs and fry for a further 2 minutes before adding the remaining spinach and beaten eggs. Season with salt and pepper. Cook over medium heat for 5 minutes, moving the mixture around a little until the sides start to set.

5. Once you can see the frittata starting to pull away a little from the pan sides, turn off the heat and place under the grill for about 5 minutes. The egg will puff up a little and the top should turn a golden colour.

6. Serve scattered with lemon zest and grated Parmesan.

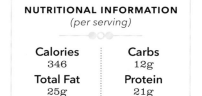

NUTRITIONAL INFORMATION
(per serving)

Calories	Carbs
346	12g
Total Fat	**Protein**
25g	21g

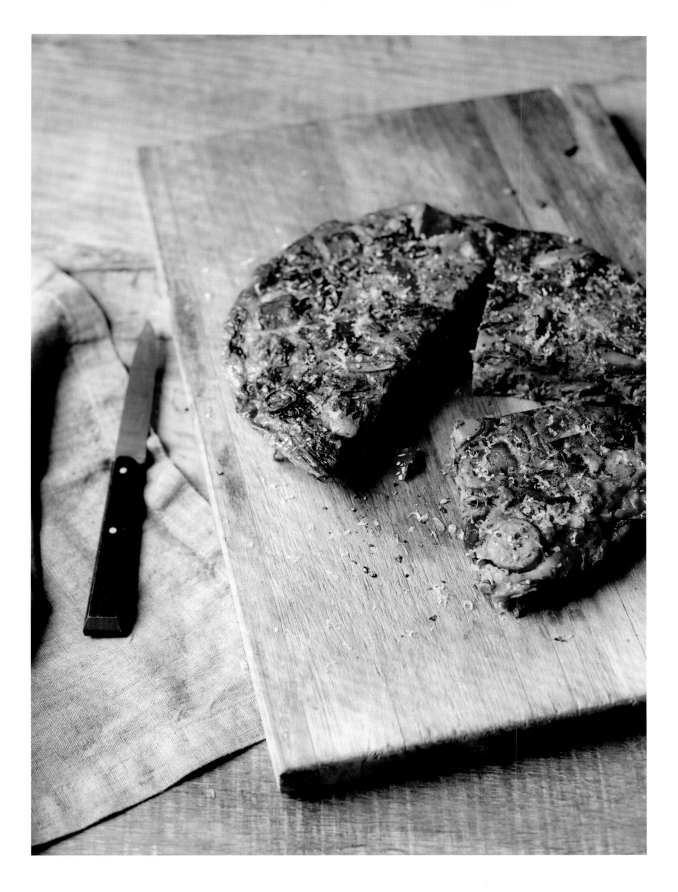

English breakfast muffins

Breakfast is the most important meal of the day – I'm sure you have heard it said a hundred times before, but I can assure you, it is true. It fills you up, gets you going, gives you energy and keeps your mind focused.

These English breakfast muffins are quick to make, extremely low in carbs, laden with good fats, protein, essential vitamins and nutrients and all the flavours work beautifully together. They are fun for kids to make, and can be enjoyed hot or cold, making them perfect for lunchboxes, picnics or a snack.

 MAKES 12 (2 PER PERSON)   **10 MINS**   **20–25 MINS**

5 rindless unsmoked back bacon rashers, cut into thin (about 1cm wide) strips

1 tsp coconut oil or use butter or olive oil, plus extra for greasing (if needed)

60g button mushrooms, thinly sliced

110g cherry tomatoes, halved

8 large eggs, beaten with 3 tbsp water

2 spring onions, finely chopped (about 30g)

sea salt and cracked black pepper

1. Preheat the oven to 200°C/400°F/gas mark 6 and grease a 12-hole muffin tin or fill it with paper cases.

2. Place a non-stick frying pan over high heat and dry-fry the bacon for about 2 minutes on each side – you want it to be cooked but not crisp as it will crisp up in the oven later. Remove from the pan and set aside.

3. Add the oil or butter to the same frying pan and fry the mushrooms for about 2 minutes, just to soften them. Set aside.

4. Place about 4 pieces of bacon into each of the 12 holes or cases in the muffin tin, followed by a few mushrooms and 2 cherry tomato halves, then pour the egg mixture on top. Sprinkle a little sea salt over the top and add some chopped spring onion and a little black pepper to finish.

5. Carefully transfer the muffin tin to the oven and bake for around 15 minutes. Look through the glass door to see if they have risen after this time – if they haven't, or still look a little soft, cook for a further 5 minutes then check again.

6. Once risen and firm, carefully remove from the oven and place on a wire rack, in the tin, to cool. The muffins will sink a little but should retain their shape.

7. Serve the muffins hot or cold; they will keep in the fridge in a sealed container for 3 days (if you leave the bacon out they will keep for 4 days).

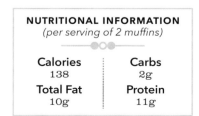

NUTRITIONAL INFORMATION
(per serving of 2 muffins)

Calories	Carbs
138	2g
Total Fat	**Protein**
10g	11g

mixed berry mini-muffin omelettes

This is one recipe that you cannot knock until you try it. It's packed with protein and is a great breakfast to grab and go. These muffins are so easy to make that you can prepare them in five minutes, pop them in the oven, have a shower and they're done. Just grab a pack of eggs, some seeds and berries and you'll be making them again, and again. With no mess and no faff, they're as delicious cold as they are straight from the oven.

MAKES 8 (2 PER PERSON)   **5 MINS**   **15 MINS**

butter or coconut oil, for greasing (if needed)

1 tbsp pumpkin seeds

1 tbsp sunflower seeds

a handful of fresh blueberries

a handful of fresh raspberries

1 tsp ground cinnamon

5 large eggs, beaten with 2 tbsp water

1. Preheat the oven to 200°C/400°F/gas mark 6 and grease 8 holes of a 12-hole muffin tin or fill with paper cases.

2. Add the seeds, berries and cinnamon to the beaten eggs and gently mix until fully combined.

3. Using a ladle or jug, divide the mixture equally among the muffin tin holes or paper cases. Cook in the oven for 15 minutes until golden brown, firm and risen.

4. Carefully remove from the oven and place on a wire rack, in the tin, to cool. Once out of the oven the muffins will sink a little, but they should retain their shape.

NOTES: Do not use frozen fruit as it will release too much water and your muffins will not rise properly.

I really recommend baking these in a silicone tray – they are heatproof and don't need greasing. If you don't have a silicone tray, grease the tin well with a little butter or coconut oil.

NUTRITIONAL INFORMATION
(per serving of 2 muffins)

Calories	Carbs
195	6g
Total Fat	**Protein**
15g	13g

raspberry muffins

A great breakfast option to eat on the go, crumbled over some Greek yoghurt, or as an afternoon tea or snack. These are delicious for the whole family and won't leave you peeling the kids from the walls! The raspberries give the muffins a delicious natural sweetness and keep them moist and moreish.

 Makes 8   **10 mins**   **20 mins**

butter or coconut oil, for greasing (if needed)

3 large eggs

100g ground almonds

50ml milk of choice (I use almond)

½ tbsp coconut flour

100g raspberries

1. Preheat the oven to 200°C/400°F/gas mark 6 and grease 8 holes of a 12-hole muffin tin or fill them with paper cases.

2. Beat the eggs and ground almonds together in a mixing bowl to a thick custard-like consistency. Add the milk and beat well with a whisk, trying to get as much air into the mixture as you can, then stir in the coconut flour. Carefully fold in all the raspberries to evenly combine.

3. Spoon the mixture into the holes of the muffin tin or the paper cases and pop into the middle of the oven and bake for 20 minutes until risen, golden and firm.

4. Carefully remove from the oven and allow to cool on a wire rack, in the tin, then serve. Alternatively, store in an airtight container in the fridge for up to 3 days.

Notes: Swap the raspberries for other fruit if you prefer, such as blackberries, blueberries or cherries.

Do not use frozen fruit in this recipe as the excess water as it defrosts would affect the consistency of the muffin.

Try adding ½ teaspoon of ground cinnamon or ground ginger.

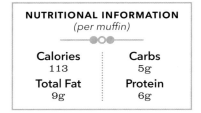

NUTRITIONAL INFORMATION
(per muffin)

Calories	Carbs
113	5g
Total Fat	**Protein**
9g	6g

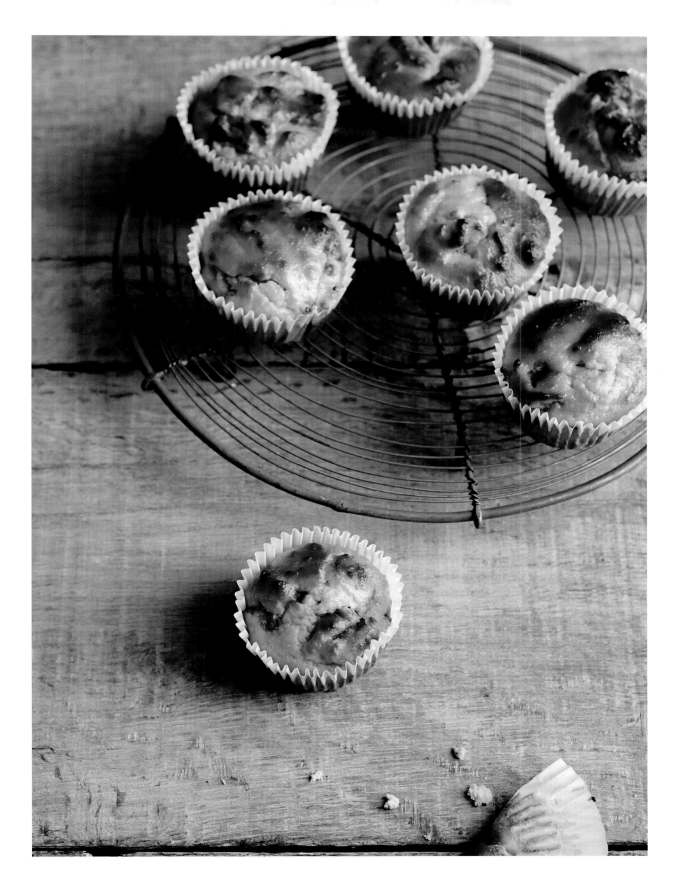

one-pan blueberry pancake

This blueberry pancake can be made in under 15 minutes. It is like a conventional pancake but without all the sugary carbs and is great for slicing up and serving with some plain or coconut yoghurt and a generous sprinkling of chopped nuts.

It's straightforward and simple, and packed with antioxidants and protein. The better quality eggs you use (free range, organic or Burford Browns), the more deliciously yellow the dish will be.

 4　 **5 MINS**　 **10–11 MINS**

2 tsp coconut oil

130g blueberries

3 large eggs, beaten with 1 tbsp water

2 tbsp coconut flour

a pinch of sea salt

a dollop of full-fat plain yoghurt and chopped nuts, to serve (optional)

1. Preheat the oven to 200°C/400°F/gas mark 6.

2. Melt the coconut oil in a large, ovenproof, non-stick frying pan over medium heat.

3. Add three-quarters of the blueberries and allow them to cook for about 3 minutes. Once they start sizzling, reduce the heat as they will spit.

4. Whisk the coconut flour and salt into the beaten eggs to form a thick custard. Pour the mixture over the blueberries, tipping the pan until the bottom is completely covered.

5. Drop in the remaining blueberries and leave for 3–4 minutes over low heat until the underside is completely cooked.

6. Once the sides have started to curl up, place the pan in the oven for about 4 minutes and cook until the top is firm.

7. Serve with a dollop of plain yoghurt and some chopped nuts, if you like.

NUTRITIONAL INFORMATION
(per serving)

Calories	Carbs
133	10g
Total Fat	**Protein**
8g	7g

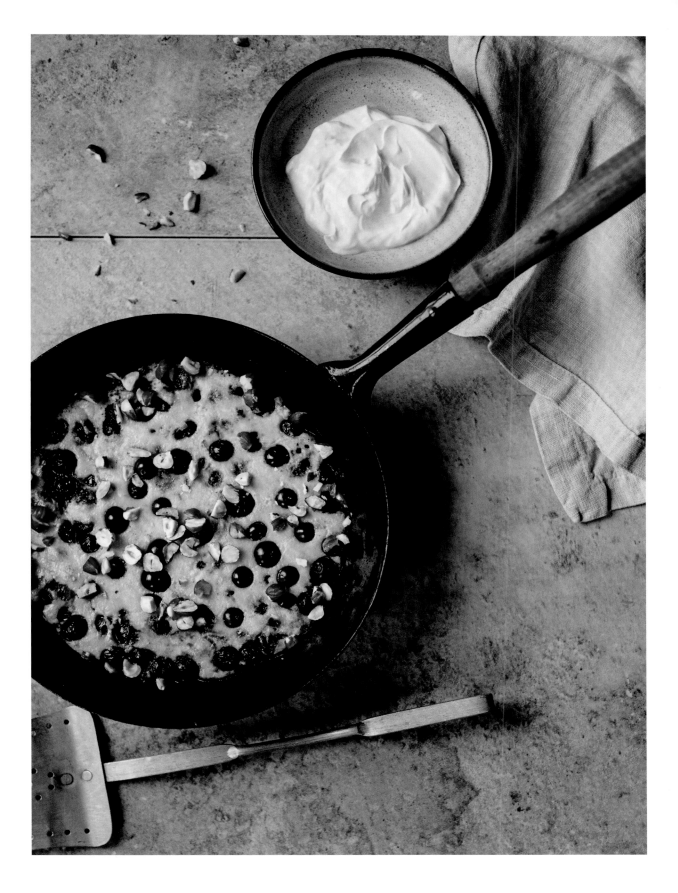

banana and peanut butter drop pancakes

With just three ingredients, these drop pancakes are incredibly easy to make and can be enjoyed hot, straight from the pan, or cold. Great for breakfast or as a snack, they are packed with protein and vitamins. I usually make six medium-sized drop pancakes and serve them with some Greek yoghurt and toasted seeds.

 2   **5 MINS**   **10 MINS**

½ banana (about 60g)

2 tsp smooth peanut butter

1 large egg, beaten

extra peanut butter, to
serve (optional)

1. Peel the banana and mash it with the peanut butter in a deep bowl until smooth and creamy with no lumps.

2. Whisk in the beaten egg and combine well. The mixture should resemble a thick custard.

3. Cook in batches of about three at a time. Add 3 x 1½ tablespoons of the mixture to a non-stick frying pan over medium heat and cook for 1½ minutes before flipping with a spatula. If the pancakes are still stuck to the pan, wait another 30 seconds before checking again. Cook on the other side for a further 1–2 minutes until cooked through. Once cooked, place them on a wire rack to cool and continue cooking the remaining batter.

4. Serve straightaway (drizzled with extra peanut butter if you wish) or allow to cool fully and store in a sealed container in the fridge until desired.

NUTRITIONAL INFORMATION
(per serving of 3 pancakes)

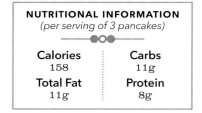

Calories	Carbs
158	11g
Total Fat	**Protein**
11g	8g

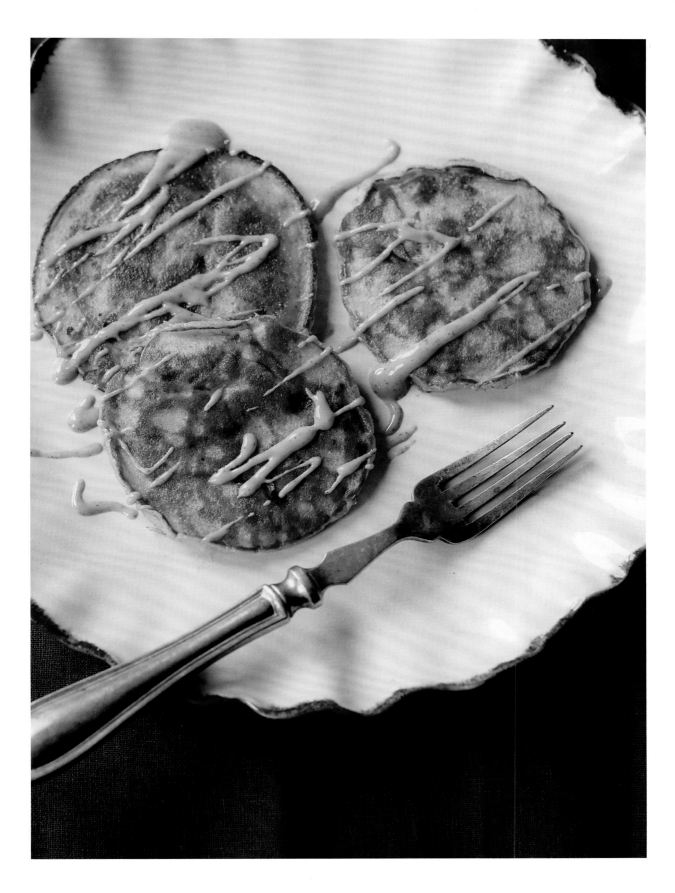

cinnamon pancakes with Greek yoghurt

These unsweetened pancakes are a delicious breakfast choice, especially for sharing with the whole family. Serve two pancakes per person, perhaps with a small handful of blueberries. Always be wary of any extras toppings as the carb content will increase and you will need to be mindful of adjusting your bolus if you are insulin dependent.

 4   10 MINS 🍲 18 MINS

2 tbsp unsalted butter, plus 2 tsp

350g almond flour (or ground almonds)

1 tbsp milled flaxseed (or crush 1 tbsp flaxseed lightly in a pestle and mortar, or pop in a coffee grinder and blitz on high speed)

½ tsp bicarbonate soda

2 tsp ground cinnamon

pinch of sea salt

3 large eggs

180ml unsweetened almond milk

4 tbsp Greek yoghurt, to serve

blueberries, to serve (optional)

1. Melt the 2 tablespoons of butter in a pan then set aside to cool a little.

2. Put the almond flour or ground almonds, flaxseed, bicarbonate of soda, cinnamon and salt in a bowl and mix thoroughly.

3. In a separate large bowl, whisk the eggs with the almond milk. Carefully whisk the melted butter into the egg mixture (it should be warm but not hot, as you do not want it to scramble the eggs!), then little by little add the flour mix, whisking continuously until it has a thick and creamy pancake-batter consistency. If it seems a little dry, add a little more almond milk, a tablespoon at a time.

4. Heat the 2 teaspoons of butter in a non-stick frying pan over a medium heat. Add about 4 tablespoons of batter (per pancake) to the pan, flattening the mixture out in the pan if it seems too thick – you should be able to to cook 2–3 pancakes at a time. The mixture makes 8 pancakes. Cook the pancakes for about 3 minutes on each side, until golden.

5. Serve them straightaway with a tablespoon of Greek yoghurt and an optional handful of blueberries.

NUTRITIONAL INFORMATION
(per serving of 2 pancakes)

Calories	Carbs
622	21g
Total Fat	**Protein**
55g	4g

Greek yoghurt with blueberry and lime jam and toasted seeds

Greek yoghurt has such a luxurious texture that it is easy to forget that it is so blood sugar-friendly. Try to opt for full-fat Greek yoghurt rather than low-fat varieties that usually contain considerable amounts of added sugar.

Combined with the sweet tartness of my homemade blueberry and lime jam, this is a truly delicious breakfast or dessert choice. If you can prepare the blueberry and lime jam the night before, this is certainly one of the quickest breakfasts you can make.

 2   **5 MINS**   **20–21 MINS**

150g blueberries

90ml water

grated zest of 1 lime and a squeeze of juice

2 tbsp mixed seeds

6 tbsp full-fat Greek yoghurt

1. First, make the jam. Place the blueberries and water in a pan over high heat, bring to the boil and cook for 2–3 minutes then reduce the heat to a simmer and cook for a further 15 minutes, stirring occasionally to ensure the fruit doesn't stick to the bottom, until all the liquid has been absorbed and the mixture has a thick jam consistency. Remove from the heat, add the lime zest and juice, then allow to cool fully before popping into a sterilised airtight jar and storing in the fridge until desired. It will keep for up to 10 days in the fridge.

2. Next, toast the seeds. Put them in a dry frying pan over medium heat and toast for 2–3 minutes until golden. Remove from the heat and set aside to cool.

3. To serve, put 3 tablespoons of Greek yoghurt into each serving bowl. Add 1 tablespoon of the blueberry jam and scatter a tablespoon of toasted seeds on top.

NUTRITIONAL INFORMATION
(per serving)

Yoghurt and seeds		*Blueberry and lime jam*	
Calories 164	**Carbs** 11g	**Calories** 22	**Carbs** 6g
Total Fat 12g	**Protein** 7g	**Total Fat** 1g	**Protein** 0.5g

NUT MILK
AND *how to* MAKE YOUR OWN

Homemade nut milks are great as they are incredibly low in carbs and packed full of goodness. Made with only two key ingredients: the nut itself and water (preferably filtered). Preservative- and additive-free nut milks are ideal for those who cannot tolerate lactose or dairy, for those who do not like milk, or for those who just want to try something different. This is a perfect way to enjoy the versatility of a protein-packed milk without the dairy proteins and added sugars from the lactose.

You can add your own spices and flavours, too, and add them to homemade granola, muffin recipes (see page 56), coffee, tea, or as a drink on their own.

Making nut milk is really easy. Simply soak the nuts in water overnight for a minimum of eight hours or for up to 48 hours – the longer you can soak them, the creamier the milk will be. Then just drain and rinse the nuts and blend them in fresh water. You will need a nut milk bag or piece of muslin to drain the blended 'milk' – set a bowl underneath to catch the nut milk, then keep the pulp, which you can dehydrate in the oven to make granola or whiz up to make almond flour (see Note on page 66).

Homemade nut milk must be stored in a sealed bottle in the fridge. It will only last a few days, so don't make too much at a time.

Here are my top nut milk recipes (you can replace any of the nuts mentioned with your nut of choice).

almond milk

I have been making almond milk for the last few years. It's delicious, fresh, creamy and perfect for those seeking an alternative to cow's milk. It is straightforward to make and you can flavour it with vanilla or cinnamon. The longer you can soak the almonds, the creamier the milk – I usually soak mine overnight.

 MAKES 1.2L (SERVES 3)   **10 MINS, PLUS AT LEAST 8 HOURS SOAKING**

150g whole almonds, skin on

1 tsp vanilla extract, or seeds scraped from 1 vanilla pod (optional)

1 litre water (preferably filtered)

1. Place the almonds in a bowl and cover with water. Leave to soak for a minimum of 8 hours.

2. Once the nuts have soaked, drain off all the water and put the almonds in a blender or food processor with the vanilla extract, if using, and the litre of water. Blitz on the highest speed for about 1 minute.

3. Use a nut milk bag or line a sieve with a piece of muslin square and set it over a bowl or jug, then pour in the nut milk mixture. Allow to drain. When most of the liquid has drained off, pick up the nut milk bag or pull up each side of the muslin and twist it together to squeeze out any remaining liquid. Tip the pulp into a separate bowl to use separately (see Note on page 66).

4. Pour the liquid into a clean, sealable glass bottle and keep in the fridge for 3 days. There will be sediment at the bottom of the bottle when you go to use it, but don't worry, just shake it up before serving.

almond milk...

NOTES: Don't throw away the almond pulp (almond meal) that is left behind. It can be used in baking (try it in bread, crackers, a quiche base or muffins) or added straight to smoothies. You can also extend its shelf life by baking it: spread it over a baking tray and pop it in the oven set to 110°C/230°F/gas mark ¼ for 2–2½ hours until toasted, stirring it occasionally to stop it browning too much. Remove from the oven and leave it to cool fully, then place in a sealed jar for baking or to use in granola, etc. Or, if you want to make almond flour, blitz it in a blender or food processor on high power to a flour-like consistency. Store in a sealed container or freeze until needed.

If you are not a big fan of almonds, or just want to try out another nut, use any of the following, substituting them in the same quantity as on the previous page. Each nut needs a minimum of 8 hours to soak, other than cashews, which only require 3 hours.

- almonds
- cashews
- hazelnuts
- macadamias
- pecans
- pine nuts
- walnuts
- pistachios
- brazil nuts

NUTRITIONAL INFORMATION
(per 100ml)

Calories	Carbs
76	1g
Total Fat	**Protein**
8g	3g

creamy cashew and cinnamon milk

A delightfully smooth drink with a hint of spice. Perfect at any time of year; served chilled with some ice straight from the blender or warmed for a comforting treat.

  MAKES 1.2L (SERVES 3)   **3 MINS, PLUS AT LEAST 3 HOURS SOAKING**

150g cashew nuts

1 tsp ground cinnamon

750ml water (preferably filtered)

1. Put the cashew nuts in a bowl and cover with water. Leave to soak for a minimum of 3 hours.

2. Once the nuts have soaked, drain all the water and place the cashews in a blender or food processor with the cinnamon and the 750ml of water – depending on the thickness you desire, add more or less water. Blitz on the highest speed for around 1 minute until really smooth and creamy.

3. Pour into clean, sealable glass bottles, seal and store in the fridge for up to 3 days.

NUTRITIONAL INFORMATION	
Calories 279	Carbs 18g
Total Fat 22g	Protein 10g

chocolate milk

This is for all the chocoholics out there who want a chocolatey pick-me-up with none of the extra sugars, sweeteners and other additives of its processed counterparts. With the health benefits of high fibre, antioxidants, vitamins and minerals, this drink is creamy, filling and gives you all the buzzy endorphins of any chocolate treat.

 2 **2 MINS**

425ml chilled Almond milk (see page 65)

½ tbsp cacao or cocoa powder

1 tbsp almond butter

1. Put the Almond milk, cacao or cocoa and almond butter in a blender and blitz on high speed for about 1 minute, until fully blended and frothy.

2. Pour straight into a glass, add a straw and enjoy!

NUTRITIONAL INFORMATION (per serving)	
Calories 92	Carbs 5g
Total Fat 8g	Protein 3g

mixed berry smoothie bowl

If you are in a rush, feeling a little under the weather, overheating in the summer sun or just want to try something new, this smoothie bowl is for you. It is a family-friendly breakfast all on its own – delicious, nutrition-packed and filling. Topped with your choice of nuts, toasted seeds, fresh berries, coconut flakes, cacao nibs or shavings of high-percentage-cocoa dark chocolate, it takes only minutes to prepare and gives you a huge boost of low-sugar nutrients and antioxidants.

Remember that despite fruit being high in fibre and vitamins, fruit sugars still have an impact on your blood sugar, so be wary of your portion size.

 2   5 MINS

250g mixed frozen blueberries and raspberries

4 tbsp full-fat Greek yoghurt

1 tbsp almond butter

juice of 1 lime

water or milk, for blending (if needed)

1. Place the frozen berries, Greek yoghurt, almond butter and lime juice in a high-powered blender, food processor or smoothie maker and blitz until smooth but thick. If it's still too thick, add a little water or milk until it reaches the desired consistency.

2. Divide the smoothie mixture between bowls and add your favourite toppings.

NOTE: Buy fruit that is on sale or in the reduced section of the supermarket, and once home, wash it and place in a sealed container in the freezer. It will retain all its nutritional goodness. Frozen berries are great eaten straight from the freezer, thawed, or popped into omelettes (see page 36) or blended into smoothies.

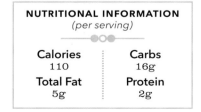

NUTRITIONAL INFORMATION
(per serving)

Calories	Carbs
110	16g
Total Fat	**Protein**
5g	2g

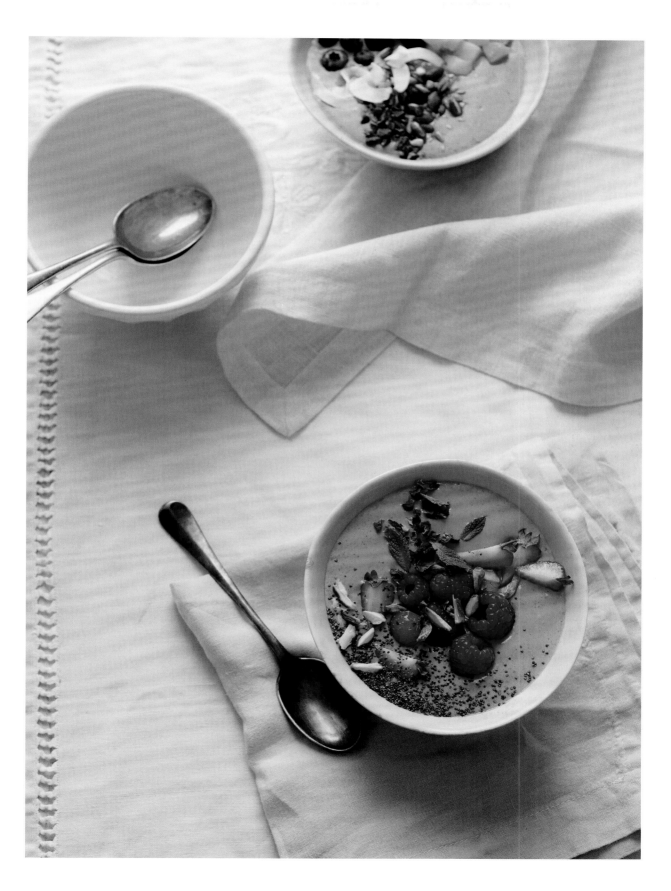

blueberry and almond butter smoothie

This blueberry and almond butter smoothie is not like your average shop-bought smoothie – made with simple ingredients, it's fresh and creamy but low in carbs and sugars. This makes it great for the whole family, especially as it won't give kids that sugar high and you can be sure that what's being consumed is natural and packed with vitamins, protein and antioxidants. Smoothies are higher in fruit sugars than egg-based breakfast dishes and therefore have an impact on your blood sugar. Be mindful of portion size.

You will need a high-powered blender, food processor or smoothie maker.

 2   5 MINS

130g blueberries
300ml almond milk
1 tbsp almond butter

1. Place all the ingredients in a high-powered blender and blitz until smooth and creamy.

2. Add more almond milk if you would like a thinner consistency.

3. Serve straightaway in a glass jar with a straw and enjoy. It's perfect for breakfast with a couple of boiled eggs.

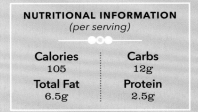

NUTRITIONAL INFORMATION
(per serving)

Calories	Carbs
105	12g
Total Fat	**Protein**
6.5g	2.5g

hazelnut chocolate spread

It's so hard to find decent sweet spreads. Most are overdosed in sugar, while the ones that are labelled 'sugar free' or 'suitable for diabetics', especially the jams, are rammed so full of sweeteners as well as the fruit's own sugar that they are not much healthier. In fact, anything that's labelled as 'suitable for diabetics' or 'sugar free' should be avoided if possible! This homemade version of a chocolate favourite is great for spreading on breads, or used as icing on cakes and in smoothies.

You will need a high-powered blender or food processor to blitz the hazelnuts into a butter. There are about 12 servings' worth of spread in this recipe, so the amount of carbs per spoon is very very low.

 Makes about 150g (serves 12)   **5 mins**

150g hazelnuts (I use blanched nuts for a creamier consistency)

2 heaped tsp cacao or cocoa powder

½ tsp seeds from 1 vanilla pod, or ¼ tsp vanilla extract

125ml almond milk or milk of choice

1. Place the hazelnuts into a food processor and blitz on highest speed for 3–4 minutes until they turn into a creamy liquid.

2. Add the cacao or cocoa powder, vanilla seeds or extract and blitz again. It will start to solidify again and crumble at this point, but keep going for 1–2 minutes.

3. Pour in the almond milk, stirring, until you get the desired consistency. It will immediately become creamy but stay thick.

4. Spoon the nut butter into a clean, sealable jar. It's best to store this in the fridge. As it does not contain high levels of sugar or preservatives, it should be consumed within 14 days.

NUTRITIONAL INFORMATION
(per serving)

Calories	Carbs
76	3g
Total Fat	**Protein**
8g	3g

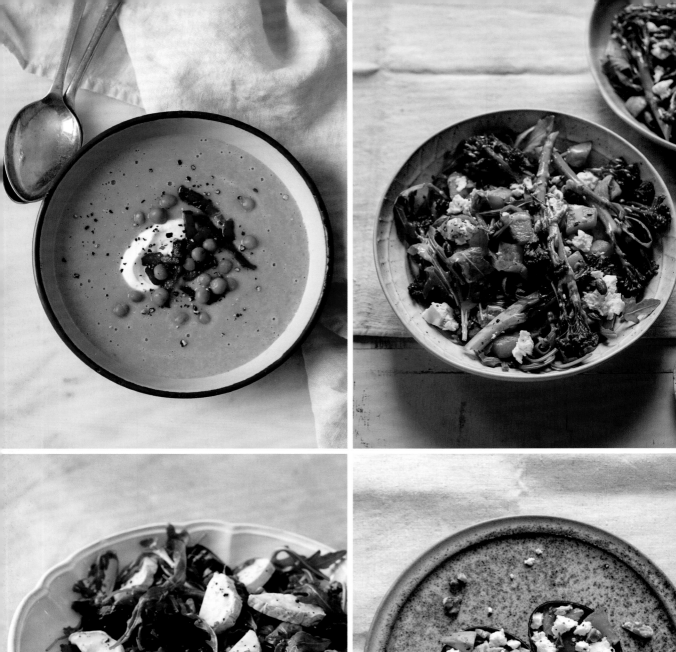
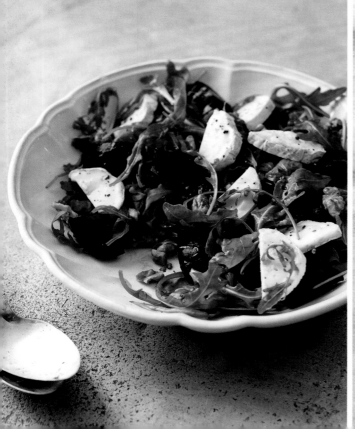
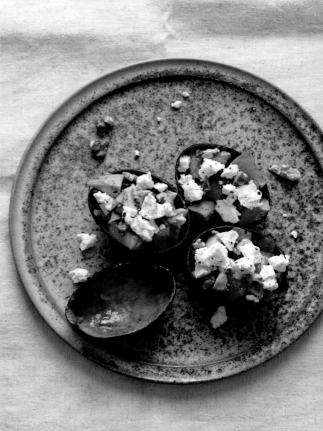

Soups & salads

───●○●───

curried carrot soup

Soup is one of the quickest dishes to make and one of the fastest ways to get a great big hit of nature's goodness inside you. This soup is indulgent and would easily serve a hungry family of four and leave enough for a bowl to take to work the next day! It's so warming and filling that there's no need for any accompaniments – other than maybe a few toasted seeds on top and a sprinkling of coriander.

 4   10 MINS   36 MINS, PLUS COOLING

2 tbsp olive oil

1 white onion (about 200g), finely chopped

3 garlic cloves, finely chopped

2 tsp curry powder

1 tsp ground cumin

1 tsp sea salt

½ tsp cracked black pepper

500g carrots, roughly chopped

750ml vegetable stock

chopped coriander, toasted seeds, full-fat Greek yoghurt, to serve

1. Heat the olive oil in a deep pan over medium heat. Add the onions and garlic and fry for about 3 minutes until soft and turning golden at the edges.

2. Add the spices, salt and pepper and fry for about 3 minutes until aromatic.

3. Add the chopped carrots to the pan. Pour over 700ml of the vegetable stock (keep the remaining 50ml for later) and bring to the boil before reducing to a simmer. Cover and cook for 20 minutes, stirring occasionally.

4. Remove the lid and cook for a further 10 minutes until the carrots are tender.

5. Remove from the heat and allow to cool for a minimum of 20 minutes, then use a hand-held blender to blitz the carrots in the stock until smooth and creamy (being careful of hot splashes). If it's too thick, add a little of the remaining stock until the soup is at the desired consistency.

6. Heat through if necessary, then serve garnished with chopped coriander or some toasted seeds and a little full-fat Greek yoghurt.

NUTRITIONAL INFORMATION
(per serving)

Calories	Carbs
135	18g
Total Fat	**Protein**
8g	2g

cashew and cumin soup

This is the perfect soup to serve in small bowls to kick off a dinner party or family gathering, or as a hearty helping for two. It's rich and indulgent. Allowing the soup to sit for 30 minutes before blending lets the ground cashews soak up a lot of the liquid and give the soup its indulgent creaminess. Once you've made this, I can assure you that you'll be making it again and again.

  4   **10 MINS**   **40 MINS, PLUS COOLING**

2 tbsp butter

1 medium onion (about 225g), diced

1 celery stick, thinly sliced

1 garlic clove, crushed

80g freshly ground cashew nuts (make this in a food processor, or by hand with a pestle and mortar, until it forms a flour-like consistency)

½ tsp ground cumin, plus a pinch to serve

¼ tsp grated nutmeg

750ml chicken stock

sea salt and cracked black pepper

1 tbsp olive oil, to serve

1. Melt the butter in a deep pan over medium heat, add the onion, celery and garlic and fry gently for 4–5 minutes until soft.

2. Add the ground cashews, cumin, nutmeg and stock and cover with a lid. Simmer over low heat for 30 minutes, stirring occasionally.

3. Remove from the heat and leave to stand at room temperature for 30 minutes (this is an important part of the process) then blitz with a hand-held blender in the pan or pop the soup into a blender and blitz until smooth.

4. Return the soup to the pan and cook over medium heat, uncovered, for 2–3 minutes until ready to serve.

5. Add salt and pepper to taste and serve garnished with a pinch of cumin and swirl of the olive oil.

NOTE: If you are using homemade chicken stock (see page 129) add salt to taste at the end, but if you are using a chicken stock cube you shouldn't need more salt.

NUTRITIONAL INFORMATION
(per serving)

Calories	Carbs
209	14g
Total Fat	**Protein**
17g	6g

beetroot and coconut soup

Here's a subtle but flavourful soup, which is warming, substantial and gives you a jolly big dose of vitamins and nutrients. I always recommend buying fresh ingredients when you can – in this case, beetroot – but if you can't, buy pre-cooked beetroot packed in its own juice (not in vinegar). This soup is very easy to make, beautifully vibrant in colour and perfect with some of my Super seed bread (see page 198).

 4   **15 MINS**   **50 MINS, PLUS COOLING**

1 tsp coconut or olive oil

3 garlic cloves, finely chopped

1 red onion (about 250g)

2 tsp paprika

2 tsp ground cumin

550g raw uncooked beetroot (about 3), peeled and cut into 5mm cubes (or use pre-cooked beetroot)

600ml vegetable stock

1 tsp each sea salt and cracked black pepper

1 x 400ml tin coconut milk

1. Heat the coconut oil in a deep pan over high heat. Add the garlic and onion and fry for 2–3 minutes until soft and golden brown.

2. Stir in the spices and continue to fry for 2–3 minutes, stirring with a wooden spoon. Add the beetroot cubes and fully coat them in the mixture in the pan, then fry for further 3 minutes. If you're using pre-cooked cubed beetroot, add them now. Pour in the stock, season with the salt and pepper and bring to the boil for a few minutes before reducing to a simmer and simmering for 40 minutes or until the beetroot is tender and cooked through (or just 10 minutes if using pre-cooked beetroot).

3. Remove from the heat and allow to cool for a minimum of 20 minutes, then carefully blitz the soup with a hand-held blender until smooth.

4. Return to the pan to the hob over low heat and add the coconut milk. Have a taste and add more seasoning if you like.

5. Serve straightaway, with my Super seed bread (see page 198) if you like, freeze or leave in the fridge for up to 5 days in an airtight container (the flavours get better the longer you leave it).

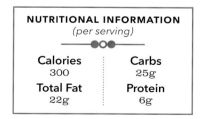

NUTRITIONAL INFORMATION *(per serving)*	
Calories 300	Carbs 25g
Total Fat 22g	Protein 6g

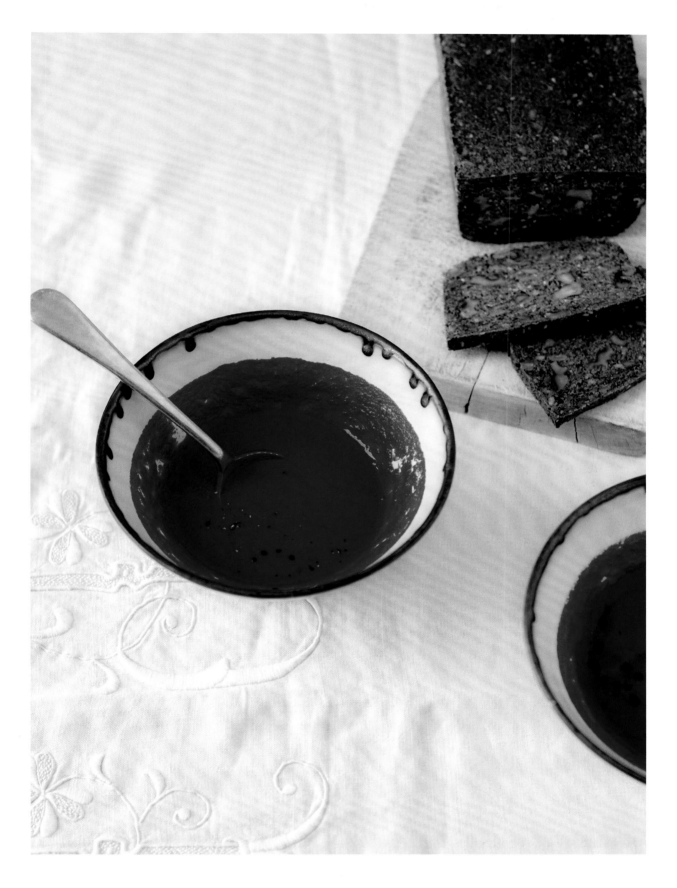

cauliflower and cumin soup

Comfort in a bowl. A simple yet tasty alternative to a potato-based soup.
Cauliflower is an underrated vegetable and this soup proves it can be
enjoyed in a variety of different ways. This is a smooth, thick, creamy and
filling soup that takes very little time to make and is perfect with a couple
of slices of buttered bread (see page 198). Filled with only natural, health-
boosting and blood sugar-friendly ingredients, it is jam-packed with flavour.

 4   10 MINS   26 MINS, PLUS COOLING

1 tbsp olive oil

1 onion (190g), finely
diced

1 garlic clove, thinly sliced

2 tsp ground cumin, plus
extra to serve

1 tsp sea salt and a pinch
of pepper

¼ tsp grated nutmeg

550g cauliflower, cut into
florets and tough stalks
removed

750ml chicken or
vegetable stock

150ml coconut milk

toasted flaked almonds,
to serve

1. Heat the oil in a deep, heavy-based pan over medium
heat. Add the onion and garlic and fry for 3–4 minutes,
until softened. Add the cumin, salt, pepper and nutmeg
and fry for a further 1–2 minutes, until fragrant. Tip in
the cauliflower and pour in the stock. Bring the mixture
to the boil, then reduce the heat and simmer for about
20 minutes, until the cauliflower is tender. Remove from
the heat and allow to cool for a minimum of 20 minutes.

2. Carefully pour the soup mixture into a food processor
and blend to a purée, or use a hand-held blender in the
saucepan.

3. Return the puréed soup mixture to the pan and add
the coconut milk. Season to taste with salt and pepper
and reheat when ready to serve.

4. Serve with a garnish of toasted flaked almonds and
a pinch of cumin.

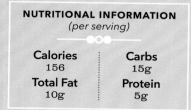

NUTRITIONAL INFORMATION
(per serving)

Calories	Carbs
156	15g
Total Fat	**Protein**
10g	5g

creamy mushroom soup

This rich, thick, smooth and creamy soup is one of my favourite go-to soups, especially on a weeknight when there's not much time for cooking. My husband and toddler both love it and it's a winning dinner-party starter, too. Incredibly low in carbs, it is quick to make and the ingredients are easy to find in your local supermarket. I like to use a mixture of mushrooms in but any standard supermarket mushroom will suffice; the cream cheese adds to the depth of flavour. I often make a double batch and freeze half.

 4   **10 MINS**   **24 MINS, PLUS COOLING**

2 tbsp olive oil

1 white onion (about 200g), finely chopped

2 garlic cloves, finely chopped

350g mushrooms, cleaned and finely sliced

600ml vegetable stock

¼ tsp grated nutmeg

2 tbsp full-fat cream cheese

150ml coconut milk

sea salt and cracked black pepper

1. Heat the olive oil in a large pan over high heat. Add the onion and sweat for 3 minutes, until softened and golden, then add the garlic and mushrooms and fry for a further 3–4 minutes until the mushrooms are soft.

2. Add the vegetable stock, bring to the boil, then reduce the heat and simmer for 15 minutes.

3. Stir in the nutmeg, cream cheese and coconut milk and cook for a further 2 minutes. Remove from the heat and allow to cool for a minimum of 20 minutes.

4. Carefully pour the soup mixture into a food processor and blend to a purée, or use a hand-held blender in the saucepan.

5. Return the puréed soup mixture to the pan and add salt and pepper to taste. Reheat when ready to serve.

NUTRITIONAL INFORMATION
(per serving)

Calories	Carbs
206	13g
Total Fat	**Protein**
17g	4g

tomato and basil soup

This rich soup is quick to make using simple ingredients, so much so that you'll never want to buy a tin of tomato soup again! I've included courgette to the otherwise classic combination of flavours, which adds to the soup's creaminess and smooth, comforting texture. You can make this in advance and freeze it, if you like, then enjoy it hot or cold.

 4   10 MINS   27 MINS, PLUS COOLING

2 tbsp olive oil

1 large white onion (about 320g), roughly chopped

3 garlic cloves, roughly chopped

1 courgette (about 200g), roughly chopped

1 chicken or vegetable stock cube

800ml chicken or vegetable stock

875g large ripe tomatoes (about 8 medium), halved

a handful of basil leaves, plus extra, chopped, to serve

1 tsp paprika

1 tsp sea salt and a pinch of cracked black pepper

full-fat plain yoghurt, to serve (optional)

1. Heat the olive oil in a large pan over high heat, then add the onion, garlic and courgette. Reduce the heat and fry for about 7 minutes until soft.

2. Add the tomatoes to the onions and courgette, and pour in the stock. Bring to the boil then reduce to a simmer and pop the lid on. Cook for 20 minutes until the tomatoes are tender and the skins are peeling off.

3. Remove from the heat, add the basil leaves, paprika, sea salt and cracked black pepper.

4. Once cooled, using a hand-held blender or liquidiser, blitz the soup until smooth.

5. Season to taste and serve straightaway with a swirl of plain yoghurt and some chopped basil (or reheat it).

NOTE: Use the best-quality ripest tomatoes you can afford. If you grow your own tomatoes it's a great soup for using up any split or overripe ones. Unfortunately, a lot of tomatoes sold in supermarkets are hard and full of water, which will dilute any flavour in this soup.

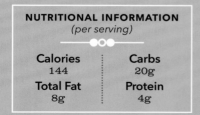

NUTRITIONAL INFORMATION
(per serving)

Calories	Carbs
144	20g
Total Fat	**Protein**
8g	4g

almonds, crunchy green vegetables and feta with a basil and garlic dressing

Whoever thought a salad could be exciting? Well, if you haven't, you will now ... This is full of taste, texture and is packed with vitamins, nutrients and healthy fats. It's an easy salad to take to work for lunch or to serve alongside a picnic, a barbecue or as a delicious side dish with a roast chicken in the summer.

Eating food that is good for you makes you feel great, and your body and blood sugars will thank you for it!

 4   10 MINS   5 MINS

For the green salad

16 French beans, trimmed

6 Tenderstem or thin-stemmed broccoli

8 asparagus spears, woody ends removed

60g almonds, chopped

4 handfuls of rocket leaves

4 spring onions (about 60g), thinly sliced

100g feta, crumbled

a pinch of sea salt

For the dressing

6 tbsp olive oil

6 basil leaves, finely chopped

1 garlic clove, crushed

juice of ½ small lemon

1. First, make the dressing. Pour the olive oil into a jug and stir in the chopped basil, crushed garlic and lemon juice. Allow to infuse for as long as possible – preferably overnight, but the longer you can leave it, the better. Keep at room temperature and sealed until required.

2. Bring a pan of water to the boil over high heat. Add the beans, broccoli and asparagus, reduce the heat to a simmer and cook for 2 minutes until tender but with some bite (al dente). Drain and pop into a bowl of iced water to stop them cooking any further and to keep their vibrant green colour.

3. Dry-toast the chopped almonds in a small pan until golden. Set aside to cool.

4. Put the rocket, beans, broccoli and asparagus into a mixing bowl and toss well, then arrange on a serving dish and top with the sliced spring onions, toasted almonds, feta and sea salt.

5. Pour the dressing evenly over the salad and serve.

NUTRITIONAL INFORMATION
(per serving)

salad		*dressing*	
Calories	Carbs	Calories	Carbs
212	12g	182	1g
Total Fat	Protein	Total Fat	Protein
16g	11g	21g	1g

pea and bacon soup

This is a vibrantly green soup (unlike the bland sludge I used to eat from the tin!) that you can prepare in advance and freeze if necessary. I usually use fresh peas that I buy from our local farmers' market, but good-quality frozen peas will also work well. Avoid overcooking the soup, as you want to retain the bright green colour and fresh taste. If you've had a joint of gammon for a Sunday roast, keep a little aside and use it in this recipe instead of the bacon. There is no need to add any extra salt as the bacon or gammon will provide all the saltiness needed. Be mindful that this soup serves six people: it is rich and indulgent so portion sizes should be smaller than usual.

 6   10 MINS   12 MINS, PLUS COOLING

200g good-quality unsmoked back bacon rashers

knob of butter

1 medium white onion (about 180g), finely chopped

800g podded peas (fresh or frozen)

900ml chicken or vegetable stock

sea salt and cracked black pepper

full-fat Greek yoghurt (optional), to serve

1. Chop 120g of the bacon rashers into fine pieces. Chop the remaining 80g into bite-sized strips.

2. In a deep pan over medium heat, melt a little of the butter, add the finely chopped bacon and cook for 1–2 minutes. Add the chopped onion and sauté for about 4 minutes until softened, stirring often. Add the peas and stock, bring to the boil, then reduce the heat and simmer for about 6 minutes until the peas are tender. Do not overcook.

3. While the peas cook, melt a little more butter in a frying pan over medium heat and sauté the remaining bacon for 1–2 minutes, turning it a few times until slightly browning and crisp. Remove from the heat and allow to cool for a minimum of 20 minutes.

4. Remove 1 tablespoon of the soft peas and set them aside. Blitz the soup in a blender or with a hand-held blender in the pan. If it's too thick, add a little extra stock or hot water. Taste the soup and season.

5. Reheat when ready to serve, then divide the soup among bowls and top with the crisp bacon pieces, the reserved peas and a swirl of Greek yoghurt, if you like.

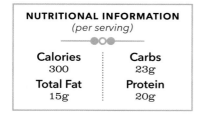

NUTRITIONAL INFORMATION *(per serving)*	
Calories 300	Carbs 23g
Total Fat 15g	Protein 20g

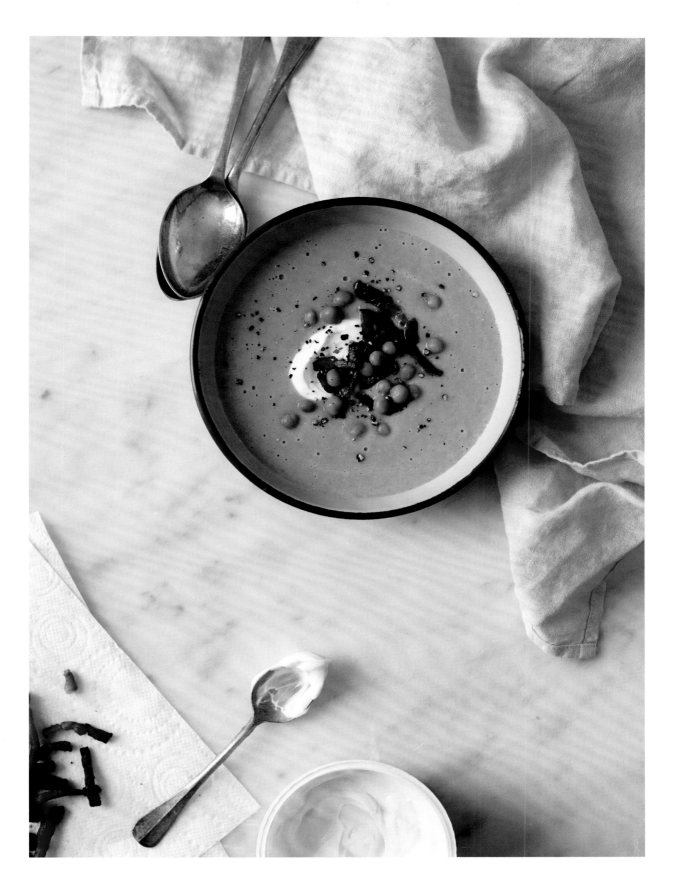

butternut squash, feta and Tenderstem salad with tahini and toasted seeds

Bright, colourful, delicious and packed with vitamins, nutrients and antioxidants, this is a dish that everyone can enjoy. Perfect for lunch or dinner, it is fresh, full of texture and abundant in taste. If required, you could reduce the amount of squash and increase the Tenderstem and rocket to decrease your carb intake.

If you would like to add more protein try some pan-fried salmon or an over-easy fried egg.

 4   **10 MINS**   **1 HOUR**

400g peeled and deseeded butternut squash, chopped into small chunks

1 tbsp olive oil

300g Tenderstem or thin-stemmed broccoli

4 tbsp mixed seeds

4 handfuls of rocket or spinach leaves

100g feta, crumbled

3 tbsp tahini paste

sea salt and cracked black pepper

1. Preheat the oven to 200°C/400°F/gas mark 6.

2. Place all the butternut squash chunks evenly on a baking sheet and drizzle with some of the olive oil. Season with salt and pepper and bake for 50 minutes until the squash is soft with browned edges.

3. Drizzle the rest of the olive oil into a wok or frying pan over high heat. Add the broccoli and stir-fry for 2–3 minutes. Add 2 tablespoons of water and cook until the water has evaporated and the broccoli is bright green and tender with browned patches. Remove and set aside.

4. Carefully wipe the pan dry with a piece of kitchen paper and place back on the heat. Tip in the mixed seeds and toast until crackling and fragrant. Set aside.

5. In 4 separate shallow bowls, put a handful of rocket or spinach followed by the roasted butternut squash, broccoli and crumbled feta. Sprinkle the toasted seeds on top and finish off with a generous drizzle of tahini.

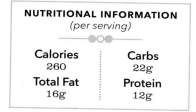

NUTRITIONAL INFORMATION	
(per serving)	
Calories	Carbs
260	22g
Total Fat	Protein
16g	12g

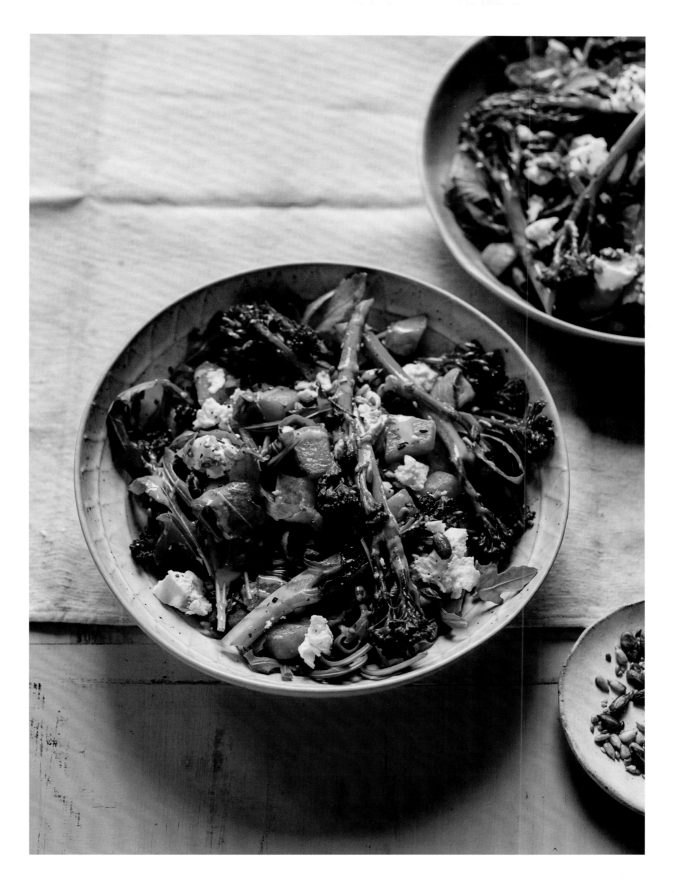

roasted aubergine and garlic salad with olive oil, basil and tomato

One of my top tips for eating well would be to never make a salad boring. A few lettuce leaves and slices of tomato just doesn't cut it. Be adventurous, mix flavours and textures. Don't dismiss the simple pleasure and all-round enjoyment you can get from a good salad.

As well as being incredibly low in carbs, this aubergine salad is divine. Aubergine is a deliciously meaty vegetable which can sometimes blend into the background, but roasted with some olive oil, sea salt, garlic and pepper it really comes alive. Combined with the vine tomatoes, pine nuts and basil, this salad is fresh, filling and simple to make.

 4   10 MINS   23–24 MINS

420g aubergine, trimmed and chopped into chunks

5 garlic cloves, roughly chopped

2 tbsp olive oil

a handful of pine nuts

230g vine tomatoes, cut into bite-sized pieces

6 basil leaves, chopped

sea salt and cracked black pepper

1. Preheat the oven to 210°C/410°F/gas mark 7.

2. Place the aubergine chunks, garlic, olive oil, salt and pepper in a mixing bowl, then toss together well, making sure all the aubergine is coated in the olive oil.

3. Spread out evenly on a baking tray and roast for 20 minutes until the aubergine is tender and browned. Remove from the oven and set aside.

4. Dry-toast the pine nuts in a pan over high heat for 3–4 minutes until they start to brown. Set aside to cool.

5. Combine the roasted aubergine, garlic, chopped tomatoes, basil and the toasted pine nuts in a bowl and serve immediately.

NUTRITIONAL INFORMATION
(per serving)

Calories	Carbs
329	15g
Total Fat	**Protein**
32g	1g

avocado stuffed with pear, feta and walnut

This is a great side dish or light lunch option. The combination of sweet, creamy, savoury and crunch work very well together and the avocado shells double up as an excellent serving bowls.

    If you'd rather leave out the pear to reduce the carbs, substitute it with cucumber or strawberries to keep the dish light and fresh.

 4   5 MINS   4–5 MINS

2 large ripe avocados, halved, de-stoned, flesh scooped out (keep the shells intact)

a handful of walnuts, chopped

knob of butter

2 ripe pears, trimmed and cut into small chunks

100g feta, crumbled

1. Chop the avocado flesh, place it in a bowl and set aside.

2. Dry-toast the walnuts in a pan over medium-high heat for 1 minute until golden and toasted. Set aside.

3. Melt the butter in the same pan over medium heat. Add the chunks of pear and sauté for 3–4 minutes until browned at the edges and caramelised.

4. Add the toasted walnuts and caramelised pear to the avocado. Carefully mix together.

5. Tip the mixture into the 4 avocado shells, then sprinkle the crumbled feta on top and serve.

NUTRITIONAL INFORMATION
(per serving)

Calories	Carbs
348	24g
Total Fat	**Protein**
28g	7g

roasted beetroot, goat's cheese and walnut salad

Sweet beetroot, toasted walnuts and goat's cheese combine beautifully in this easy salad that will not fail to impress. It has flavour and texture in every mouthful and is full of vitamins and protein. Use pre-cooked beetroot packed in its own juice (not in vinegar) instead of roasting your own, if you're short on time.

My favourite way to serve this is alongside a couple of other salad platters, with some fresh bread (see page 198) and perhaps my Roasted cod and chorizo fishcakes (see page 102). Cook this at the weekend for friends and family or store it in a sealed container to eat during the week with some fish or chicken.

 4   **15 MINS**   **1 HOUR 20 MINS, PLUS COOLING**

2 large beetroots (500g), trimmed

80g walnuts, chopped

2 handfuls of rocket leaves

1 tbsp olive oil

75g goat's cheese, cut into chunks

1. Preheat the oven to 220°C/425°F/gas mark 7.

2. Wrap the whole beetroots separately in tin foil and place on a baking tray. Roast for 1 hour 20 minutes until soft – you should be able to slide a sharp knife into them without much resistance. Remove from the oven and leave to cool for about 40 minutes, then peel off their skins by gently brushing your thumb over them in a circular motion, pulling away the skin as you go.

3. While the beetroots are cooling, dry-toast the chopped walnuts for about 1 minute in a pan over high heat until golden brown and aromatic. Set aside to cool.

4. Roughly chop or slice the beetroots into bite-sized chunks.

5. Place the rocket, half the toasted walnuts, beetroots and the olive oil in a serving dish. Toss everything together.

6. Evenly scatter over the goat's cheese and the rest of the toasted walnuts, then serve straightaway.

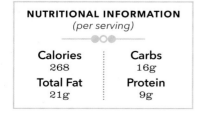

NUTRITIONAL INFORMATION
(per serving)

Calories	Carbs
268	16g
Total Fat	**Protein**
21g	9g

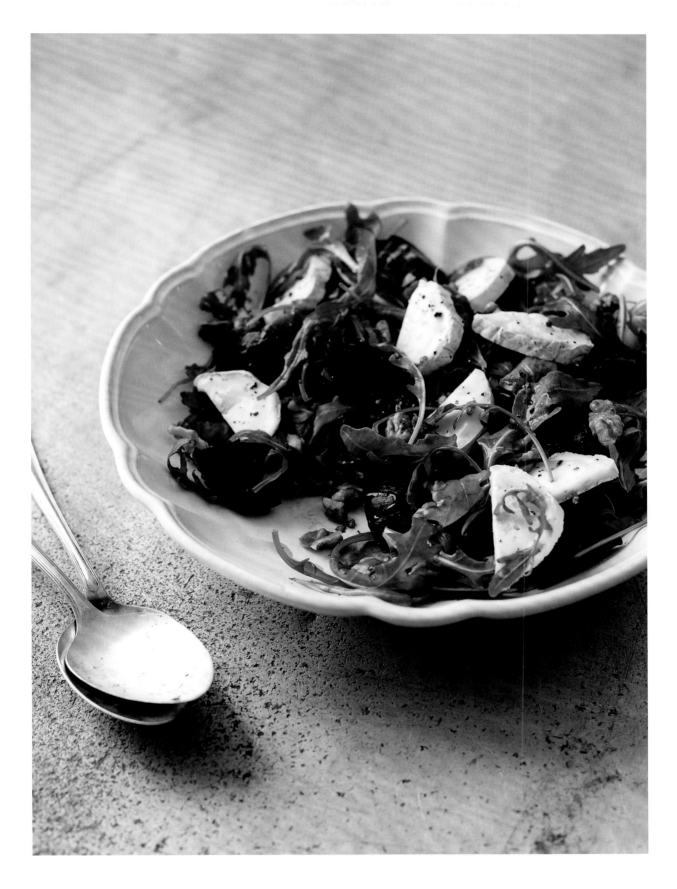

roasted Mediterranean vegetable couscous

This isn't true couscous, as it doesn't have the same stodginess. Consistency-wise it's the same and taste-wise, it's better (in my opinion). It won't leave you bloated, it won't take your blood sugar on a rollercoaster but it *will* keep you feeling full. It's the perfect accompaniment to fish or meat or as a side dish for a summer picnic or barbecue. It can be served hot or cold and is easily transportable.

6   **20 MINS**   **35–40 MINS, PLUS COOLING**

100g baby plum tomatoes (or any baby tomatoes you can get your hands on!)

215g red pepper, deseeded and roughly chopped

200g red onion, roughly chopped

100g courgette, chopped

100g aubergine, thickly sliced and halved or quartered

2 garlic cloves, diced

1 tbsp olive oil, plus extra for drizzling

450g cauliflower, cut into florets, tough stalks removed

knob of butter

squeeze of lemon

a handful of pomegranate seeds

a handful of coriander leaves

sea salt and cracked black pepper

1. Preheat the oven to 200°C/400°F/gas mark 6.

2. Place all the vegetables, including the garlic, in a bowl with the olive oil and some sea salt, toss until the veg are all coated, then tip onto a baking sheet and pop in the oven to roast for 35–40 minutes.

3. While the vegetables are cooking, make the cauliflower rice. Blitz the cauliflower in a food processor until it has a rice-like consistency. Alternatively, use a box grater to grate the cauliflower by hand. Put the grated cauliflower in a piece of muslin, or a sieve lined with kitchen paper set over a bowl and allow all the water to drain away.

4. Melt the butter in a pan over low heat. Add the cauliflower rice and a pinch of salt and cook, stirring occasionally, for 4–5 minutes until it has softened but still retains its bite.

5. Turn off the heat and tip the cauliflower into a serving bowl to cool.

6. Remove the roasted vegetables from the oven and allow them to cool for about 20 minutes or so before adding them to the couscous.

7. Add a generous squeeze of lemon, drizzle of olive oil, sprinkle of pepper, the pomegranate seeds and coriander. Serve warm or cold and enjoy with a little protein if you desire, such as chicken or baked salmon.

NUTRITIONAL INFORMATION
(per serving)

Calories	Carbs
93	17g
Total Fat	**Protein**
3g	3g

pan-fried sprouts with orange, chorizo and hazelnuts

This is a recipe I have made for lots of guests over the years and one that has converted even the biggest sprout hater (and let me tell you, there are quite a few), into a sprout lover. The trick lies in the flavour and texture, and it's important not to overcook them. Never boil a sprout, always wok- or pan-fry it and add the right ingredients for a super-nutritious, divine-tasting and blood sugar-friendly bowl of goodness. The contrast of the sprouts with the tartness of the orange, the saltiness of the chorizo and crunch of the hazelnuts works beautifully. It's comforting, filling and incredibly moreish, with nothing to feel guilty about.

This recipe works well as a side dish, especially throughout the colder winter months.

 4   **5** MINS   **12** MINS

1 tsp coconut oil

1 medium red onion (about 225g), chopped

12cm chunk of chorizo, chopped into bite-sized pieces (remove any papery skin from the chorizo)

400g Brussels sprouts, halved

125ml water

150g spring greens or kale, chopped into bite-sized pieces

80g hazelnuts, chopped in half (or you can use 50g each of pumpkin seeds/ sesame seeds/flaked almonds)

a pinch of sea salt

2 tsp grated orange zest

1. Melt the coconut oil in a deep wok, then add the red onion and chorizo and fry for about 3 minutes until soft. Add the Brussels sprouts and fry for 3–4 minutes. Pour in the water, a little at a time, to help the sprouts cook through and stop them sticking. Add the spring greens or kale and cook together for about 2 minutes.

2. Dry-toast the chopped hazelnuts (or other nuts/ seeds), then add them to the sprout mixture. Take off the heat and add the salt and orange zest.

3. Serve immediately alongside a roasted meat of choice, or enjoy as a salad on its own. Alternatively, allow to cool then pop into an airtight container and keep in the fridge for up to 3 days.

NUTRITIONAL INFORMATION
(per serving)

Calories	Carbs
260	22g
Total Fat	**Protein**
17g	11g

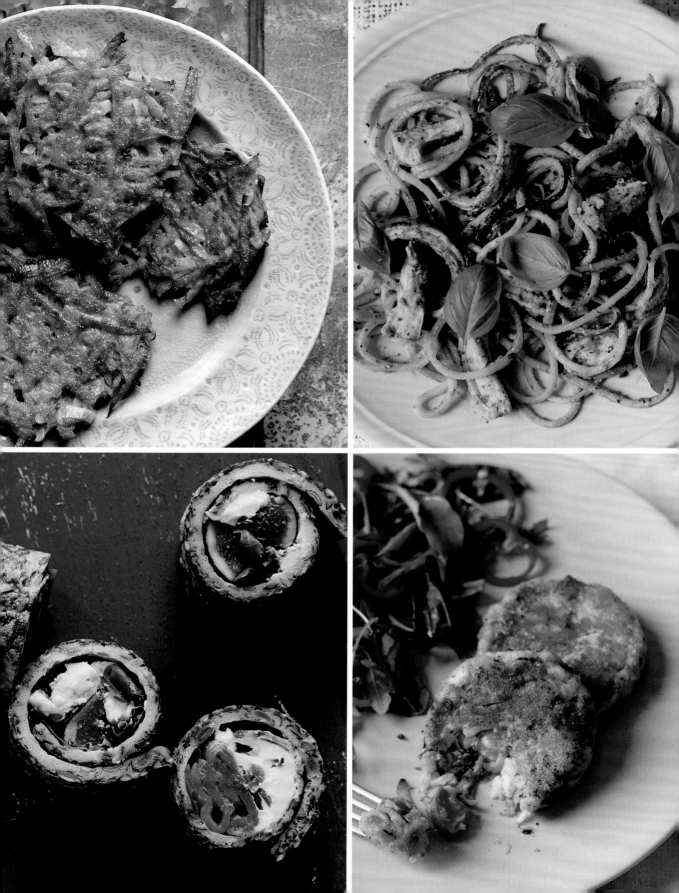

Light bites

courgette 'spaghetti' with pesto and chicken

This is a great recipe for using up the leftovers from a roast chicken (see page 128). This is a healthy, blood sugar-friendly, low-carb alternative to traditional spaghetti with pesto. An easy to make, no-fuss and no-cook courgette recipe which uses the simplest of ingredients to make the most delicious meal.

Don't knock it until you try it. I can assure you it will leave you feeling full and your taste buds more than satisfied.

 2   **15** MINS

500g courgettes

6 handfuls of basil leaves

45g pine nuts

2 large garlic cloves, peeled

a handful of rocket leaves, plus extra to garnish

1 tbsp olive oil

1 tbsp crème fraîche

150g skinless and boneless cooked chicken, shredded

sea salt

1. Using a spiralizer (see Note below), create noodles out of the courgette, or use a vegetable or julienne peeler, or a sharp knife to carefully cut the courgette into long thin strands. Place the courgette spaghetti in a big mixing bowl.

2. Blitz the basil, pine nuts, garlic, rocket and a pinch of salt in a blender or food processor. Pulse 4–5 times until well mixed and broken up. Pour the olive oil in a little at a time until the mixture is thick and creamy. You will probably have to use a spatula to scrape down the sides. Add the crème fraîche and blitz until combined.

3. Spoon the pesto over the courgette spaghetti and, using clean hands, massage it in evenly. Add the shredded chicken and toss to combine. Serve straightaway, garnished with more basil.

NOTES: If you are not using leftovers from a roast chicken, fry 150g diced chicken or chicken strips in a little olive oil over medium heat until completely cooked through.

A spiralizer is a trendy contraption that turns the humble courgette (or any other vegetable) into beautiful spaghetti-like noodles. You can pick them up relatively inexpensively, but if you don't have one you can use a vegetable peeler and peel long strips or ribbons of the courgette. Otherwise, if you have a julienne peeler, you can replicate the noodles by peeling lengthways. Alternatively, if you have great knife skills, you could cut the courgette into spaghetti strips by hand.

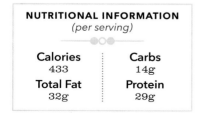

NUTRITIONAL INFORMATION	
(per serving)	
Calories	Carbs
433	14g
Total Fat	Protein
32g	29g

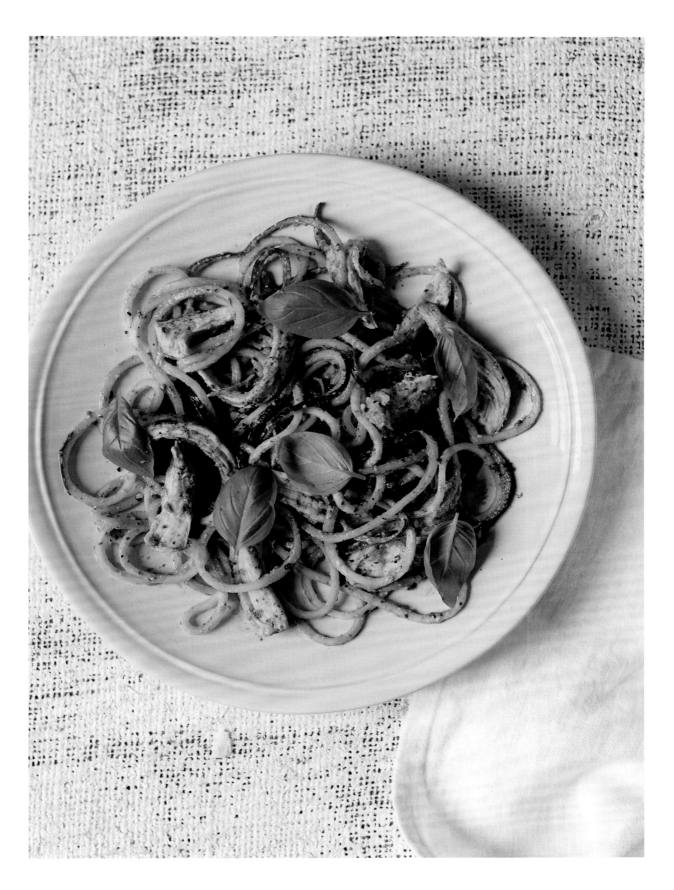

homemade coleslaw

The perfect accompaniment to a piece of salmon, this coleslaw is crunchy, light, fresh and easy to prepare in just a few minutes. It is also bright and colourful, making it a perfect centrepiece to a summer barbecue or feast with friends or family. Or, put it in a sealed container and keep it in the fridge for up to three days to jazz up other dishes. Cubes of fried chorizo or fresh feta make scrumptious additions.

 4   **10** MINS

130g cored and shredded red cabbage (you can use any cabbage you like. I use red to give the dish added vibrancy)

2 large carrots, roughly grated (145g)

150g Brussels sprouts, trimmed and roughly grated

2 spring onions (about 30g), thinly sliced

½ tsp sea salt

3 tbsp mayonnaise (see recipe on page 124)

1. Put the shredded cabbage in a mixing bowl with the grated carrots and sprouts. Add the sliced spring onions and salt.

2. With clean hands, mix the vegetables together well until evenly mixed. Add the mayonnaise and mix well with a large metal spoon until fully combined.

3. Spoon the coleslaw straight onto plates or into a beautiful serving bowl for people to help themselves.

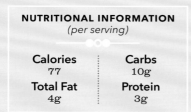

NUTRITIONAL INFORMATION	
(per serving)	
Calories	Carbs
77	10g
Total Fat	Protein
4g	3g

peppered paprika salmon

This is an easy one-pan, no-fuss weeknight meal. With only five key ingredients, it is one of the tastiest, healthiest and most foolproof dishes I cook. The whole process takes only 25 minutes from pan to plate, which is perfect for those seeking a quick, low-carb meal.

Salmon is rich in lots of nutritious health-boosting goodness. Once baked, it's filling, moist and tender, and with just a few simple additions can make for the most delicious of dishes.

It is simple to serve and just as good cold as it is hot.

 2 **5 MINS** **20 MINS**

3 tbsp olive oil

grated zest of ½ lemon

2 garlic cloves, finely chopped

1 tbsp smoked paprika

2 salmon steaks (about 175g each)

sea salt and ½ tbsp cracked black pepper

1. Preheat the oven to 210°C/410°F/gas mark 7.

2. Combine the olive oil, lemon zest, garlic and smoked paprika in a mixing bowl.

3. Place the salmon fillets skin-side down on a large piece of foil. Spoon the paprika mixture evenly over each fillet, ensuring that all parts of the fish are covered.

4. Season each fillet with salt, then sprinkle over the pepper. Wrap the foil around the fish fillets, making sure all the edges are tightly sealed.

5. Carefully place the foil package onto a baking tray in the middle of the oven and bake for 20 minutes until the fish can be easily flaked with a fork and is cooked through. Serve straightaway.

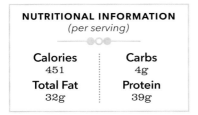

NUTRITIONAL INFORMATION
(per serving)

Calories	Carbs
451	4g
Total Fat	**Protein**
32g	39g

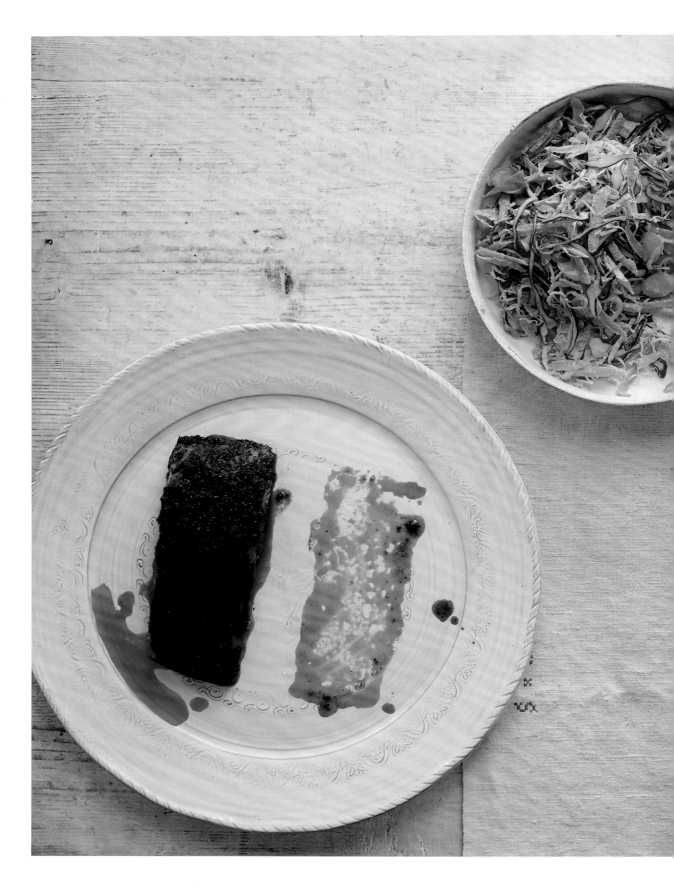

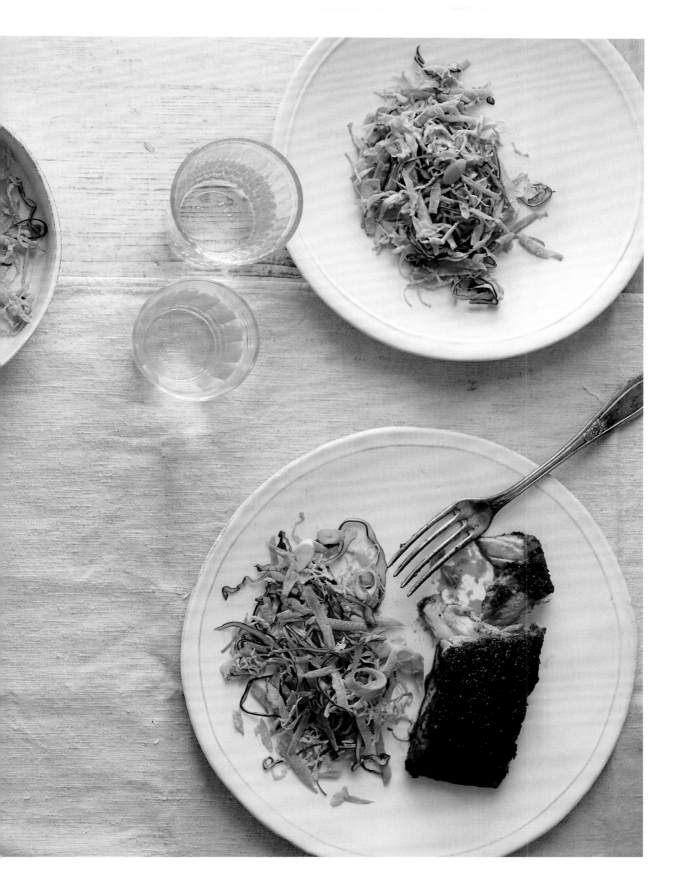

tomato, basil and mozzarella salad
with pan-fried mackerel

Succulent and tasty mackerel fillets with a beautifully crisp skin, combined with a fresh salad of tomato, basil and creamy mozzarella, make a delicious and quick meal. Mackerel is a sustainable fish and fillets are widely available, good value, take very little time to cook and are a great midweek dinner option. A little goes a long way, too, as the fish is rich and oily and jam-packed with goodness, being full of omega-3.

 4   **5 MINS**   **4–5 MINS**

a handful of basil leaves

2 handfuls of rocket leaves

2 beef tomatoes, sliced (about 300g)

1 x 220g packet of fresh mozzarella, sliced

4 mackerel fillets (about 580g total)

1 tbsp olive oil

1 garlic clove

sea salt and cracked black pepper

1. Divide the basil and rocket leaves evenly among 4 plates, then top with the tomato and mozzarella slices.

2. Slash the skin side of the fish fillets with a sharp knife and season them with salt and pepper.

3. Heat the oil in a frying pan, fry the garlic for 1 minute until slightly golden brown then remove. Add the fish, skin-side down. As the fillets curl up away from the heat, gently apply pressure to the fillets with a spatula to ensure that they stay flat and all of the skin comes into contact with the pan.

4. Once the skin is crisp and golden, turn the fillet over and remove the pan from the heat. Leave the mackerel in the pan to continue cooking in the residual heat for 30 seconds–1 minute.

5. Remove the fish from the pan and place on top of the salad or to the side, skin-side up.

NOTE: Mackerel can be tough and dry when overcooked, so err on the side of caution when cooking it. Leaving the skin on while cooking not only provides a crisp treat, but helps hold the fillet together and keep the flesh moist.

NUTRITIONAL INFORMATION
(per serving)

Calories	Carbs
537	7g
Total Fat	**Protein**
36g	47g

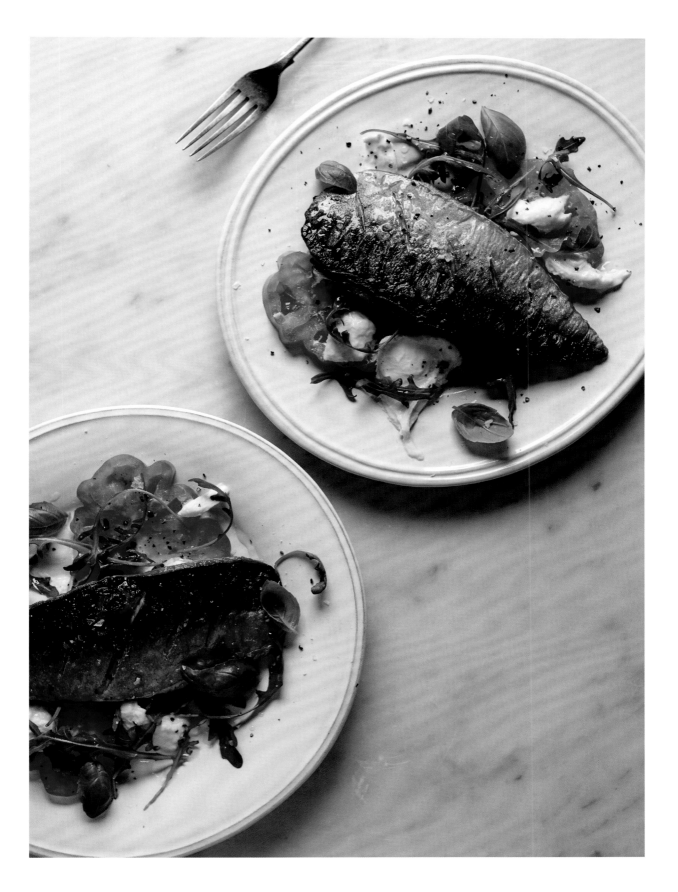

roasted cod and chorizo fishcakes

These fishcakes are succulent, full of flavour and really simple to make. Packed with omega-3 and plenty of nutritional benefits, they do more than just satisfy your taste buds.

I often make mine with cod from a local fishmonger but you can use any fish you like; I have also used trout, mackerel and salmon with successful results. The cod is meaty and moreish and the chorizo adds a beautifully salty level of deliciousness, while the sweet potato helps to bulk the cakes out and add a comforting texture.

 4   **30 MINS**   **25–27 MINS, PLUS CHILLING**

1 sweet potato (about 265g), peeled and chopped

2 garlic cloves

300g cod fillets, skin on

5 tbsp olive oil, plus extra for greasing

5cm chunk of chorizo, skin removed, chopped into bite-sized pieces

about 10 coriander leaves, chopped

1 courgette (about 190g), grated

grated zest of 1 lime, plus 1 tbsp juice

50g ground almonds, for dusting

sea salt and cracked black pepper

1. Preheat the oven to 200°C/400°F/gas mark 6.

2. Cook the sweet potato in a pan of boiling water for about 20 minutes until tender. Drain, then mash well. Set aside.

3. Place the garlic cloves and cod in a deep, well-greased roasting tray, drizzle with 1 tablespoon of the olive oil and sprinkle over some salt. Roast for 12–15 minutes until the fish is cooked through and flaking. Once cool, remove the skin and flake the fish.

4. Thinly slice the cooked garlic and set aside.

5. In a large mixing bowl, combine the mashed sweet potato, flaked cod, sliced garlic, chorizo, chopped coriander, grated courgette and lime zest and juice, season with salt and pepper and mix thoroughly.

6. Mould the mixture into 8 burger shapes with your hands. Dust them with ground almonds on all sides and place in the fridge for 1½ hours to chill and set.

7. Heat the remaining olive oil in a large frying pan over very high heat, then add the fishcakes and fry for 5–7 minutes on each side until golden brown (in batches if necessary).

8. Serve immediately with a side salad, or cool and keep in a sealed container in the fridge for later.

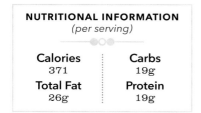

NUTRITIONAL INFORMATION
(per serving)

Calories	Carbs
371	19g
Total Fat	**Protein**
26g	19g

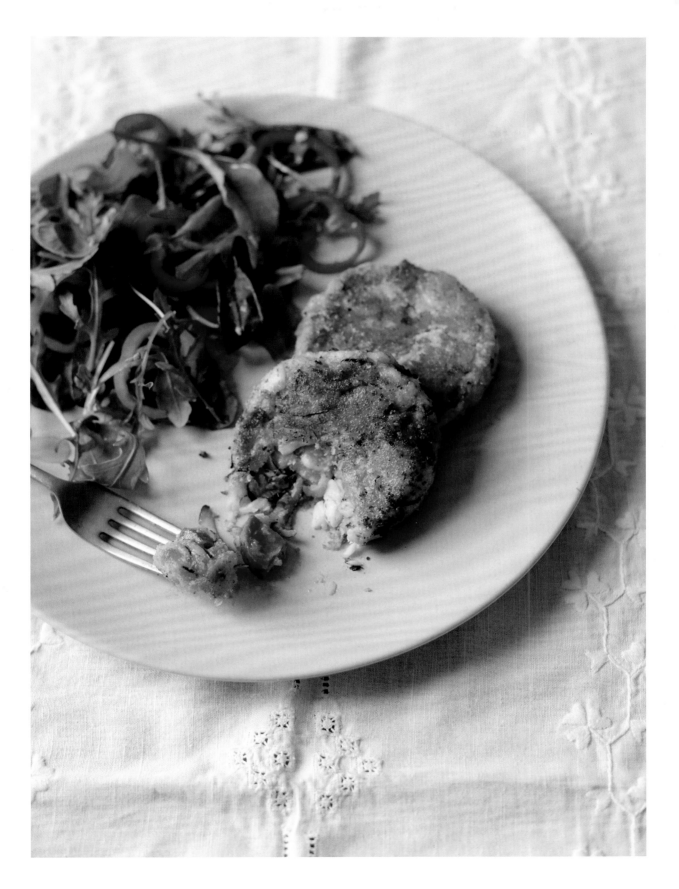

mixed fish skewers with a spicy nut butter dip

These meaty fish skewers are perfect for any season. Whether you are dining al fresco or cosying up in front of the fire, this dish oozes taste and comfort. Marinated in a blend of fresh herbs and spices, the fish chunks can be grilled, chargrilled or cooked on the barbecue. They are so easy to make and full of health-boosting goodness and the creamy dip for dunking the skewers into or drizzling over the top will go down a treat.

 4 **15** MINS, PLUS **30** MINS MARINATING **8–10** MINS

For the skewers

60ml olive oil

juice of 1 lemon

3 tbsp finely chopped
 flat-leaf parsley, plus extra
 for garnish

2 garlic cloves, crushed

1 tsp paprika

1 tsp sea salt

600g cod and salmon
 fillets, skinned and cut into
 4cm cubes

For the spicy nut
 butter dip

2 tbsp almond butter

220ml coconut milk

½ tsp each of sea salt and
 cracked black pepper

¼ tsp ground cumin

½ tsp cayenne pepper (or
 to taste)

1. Whisk the olive oil, lemon juice, parsley, crushed garlic, paprika and salt together in a small bowl. Put the fish chunks in a flat dish and pour over the marinade to evenly coat, then spread the chunks out, cover with cling film and pop into the fridge to marinate for about 30 minutes. Soak wooden skewers in cold water during this time, if using.

2. While the fish is marinating, make the spicy nut butter dip. Put the almond butter and coconut milk in a pan over medium heat, bring to the boil and simmer for 1–2 minutes, until the mixture thickens. Stir often and don't take your eye off it as you do not want it to burn. Stir in the salt, pepper, cumin and cayenne, then set aside and allow to cool. Preheat the grill about 15 minutes before you remove the fish from the fridge.

3. Push the fish chunks onto 4 separate skewers, alternating cod with salmon. Grill the fish for 4–5 minutes, then turn and grill for a further 4–5 minutes until the edges are golden and the fish is cooked through. Cut one of the chunks in half to check it's piping hot – there should be no transparent flesh. Garnish the skewers with parsley and serve with the dip alongside in a small serving pot or drizzled evenly over each of the fish skewers. Store any leftover dip in a sealed container in the fridge for up to 1 week.

NOTES: Source sustainable fish if possible.

 If you would rather cook on a griddle pan or barbecue, follow the same process – you may just need to reduce the cooking time.

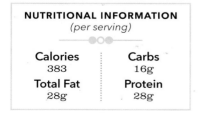

NUTRITIONAL INFORMATION	
(per serving)	
Calories	Carbs
383	16g
Total Fat	Protein
28g	28g

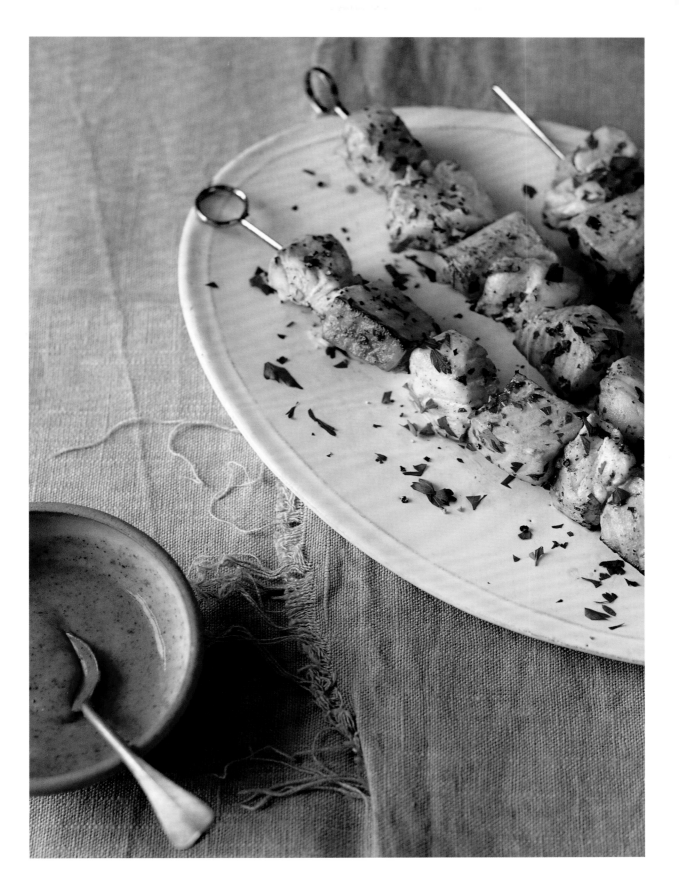

baked chicken tikka pieces

Delicious eaten hot or cold, these bites have the wonderful qualities of a chicken tikka curry with all its warmth, spice and creaminess. This recipe makes enough spice mix to fill a small jar, so you have plenty left over for other meals, such as the Coconut chicken tikka on page 132.

These chicken pieces are really easy to make and require hardly any preparation. They are also blood sugar-friendly and packed with protein and flavour. One for the whole family.

 4   10 MINS   30 MINS

450g skinless and boneless chicken breast, diced
250g full-fat Greek yoghurt
1 tsp sea salt
cracked black pepper

For the tikka spice mix
3 tsp ground coriander
3 tsp ground cumin
4 tsp paprika
2 tsp garam masala
1½ tsp ground ginger
1 tsp chilli powder

1. Preheat the oven to 220°C/425°F/gas mark 7.

2. First, make the tikka spice mix. Put all the ingredients in a clean jar, seal and shake to combine.

3. Place the chicken pieces, yoghurt, 3 heaped teaspoons of the tikka spice, the sea salt and a generous twist of cracked black pepper into a baking dish and mix well, making sure you coat all the chicken in the yoghurt and spice mixture. Spread the chicken out in the dish and bake in the oven for 30 minutes. To check the chicken is cooked, cut the largest piece of chicken in half – if any pink flesh remains, pop it back in the oven for a few minutes, until cooked through.

4. Remove from the oven and serve immediately or allow to cool fully then store in a sealed container in the fridge and eat within 2 days.

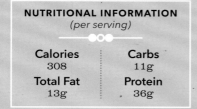

NUTRITIONAL INFORMATION
(per serving)

Calories	Carbs
308	11g
Total Fat	**Protein**
13g	36g

spinach, onion, bacon and feta quiche

Finding a quiche that is not full of blood sugar-raising ingredients is very hard. However, this recipe is low carb and full of healthy fats and lots of protein. It's perfect served hot or cold; for a lunch or picnic, it's one to slice up and share.

 6   25 MINS, PLUS 30 MINS CHILLING   40 MINS, PLUS COOLING

170g ground almonds

30g coconut flour

1 tsp dried basil

1 tsp fennel seeds

1 tsp sea salt

¼ tsp cracked black pepper

1 large egg, beaten

50g coconut oil, melted, plus extra for greasing

For the filling

1 tsp coconut oil or butter

200g red onion or white onion, chopped

3 rashers unsmoked back bacon, cut into small strips

250g spinach

3 large eggs

170ml coconut milk

1 tsp sea salt

100g feta, crumbled

½ tsp cracked black pepper

1. Preheat the oven to 200°C/400°F/gas mark 6 and grease a springform 30cm pie dish.

2. Mix the ground almonds, coconut flour, dried basil, fennel seeds, salt and pepper in a large bowl. Make a well in the middle, add the egg and fold it into the mix – the mix will become quite crumbly – then add the melted coconut oil and mix until they start to bind together. Add 3 tablespoons of cold water, one at a time, until a dough has formed. Wrap the dough in cling film and chill it for 30 minutes.

3. While the dough is chilling, prepare the filling. Melt the coconut oil or butter in a deep pan over high heat, add the onion and bacon and cook for 3–4 minutes until the onion has softened, then add the spinach and cook for 1–2 minutes until wilted. Turn off the heat and allow to cool for 10–15 minutes.

4. Roll out the chilled pastry and line the pie dish. Prick the base of the pastry with a fork or line the pie dish with greaseproof paper and fill with baking beans then blind-bake it in the oven for 10 minutes. Remove the pie crust from the oven – it might have shrunk a little and pulled away from the sides of the pie dish; this is fine!

5. While the pastry is blind-baking, continue with the filling. Whisk the eggs and coconut milk together in a large bowl then add the salt. Stir in the cooled onion, bacon and spinach mix to combine.

6. Pour the mixture into the pastry case, scatter the feta and cracked black pepper on top and bake for about 25 minutes until golden brown and set.

7. Remove from the oven and serve hot or allow to cool and keep covered in the fridge for up to 4 days.

NUTRITIONAL INFORMATION *(per serving)*	
Calories 440	Carbs 15g
Total Fat 38g	Protein 17g

pesto and Parma ham pizza

This is a one-pan recipe that is ever so simple to make and one of the lowest-carb pizza recipes you are ever likely to find! It is one recipe that will certainly get your taste buds talking, a pesto-flavoured pizza base with delicious gooey cheese on top. It tastes so naughty, but when you look at the ingredients you realise it's only full of natural goodness. And at the end of the day, anything this green has to be good, right?!

I usually slice it up for eating on the go – it's packed with far more flavour than your usual cheese sandwich.

 4   **15 MINS**   **15 MINS**

For the pesto
50g spinach leaves

30g basil leaves, plus extra to serve

50g shelled unsalted pistachio nuts

1 garlic clove, peeled

1 tsp sea salt

2 tbsp extra-virgin olive oil

For the pizza
2 tbsp water

3 large eggs, beaten

15g coconut flour

100g grated mozzarella

4 Parma ham slices

6 baby tomatoes, halved

cracked black pepper

1. Preheat the grill, or if you have an ovenproof frying pan, preheat the oven to 200°C/400°F/gas mark 6.

2. First, make the pesto. Place the spinach, basil, pistachios, garlic and salt into a food processor and pulse briefly. Add the olive oil a little at a time and blitz until the mixture is thick and creamy. If it is too thick for your liking, do add a little more oil. You will probably have to use a spatula to scrape down the sides.

3. Transfer the pesto to a large bowl and add the water and eggs and beat together until fully combined. Now add the coconut flour a little at a time (you don't want any lumps!) and mix in until everything is blended together.

4. Over a medium heat, pour the mixture into a non-stick frying pan until it evenly covers the bottom of the pan (grease the pan it if it's not non-stick). Cook for 6 minutes, until you can see the edges lifting a little. You should be able to lift the pizza a little with a spatula to see if the bottom's cooking.

5. Transfer the pan to the grill or the oven and cook for 5 minutes then carefully remove the pan and scatter the mozzarella, Parma ham, tomato halves and some cracked black pepper over the pizza base. Place back under the grill or into the oven for about 3 minutes until the mozzarella is melted and golden on top and the tomatoes are softening.

6. Garnish with some basil leaves, slice up and enjoy! Alternatively, allow to cool before transferring to a plate, covering and keeping in the fridge until required.

NUTRITIONAL INFORMATION
(per serving)

Calories	Carbs
312	9g
Total Fat	**Protein**
23g	19g

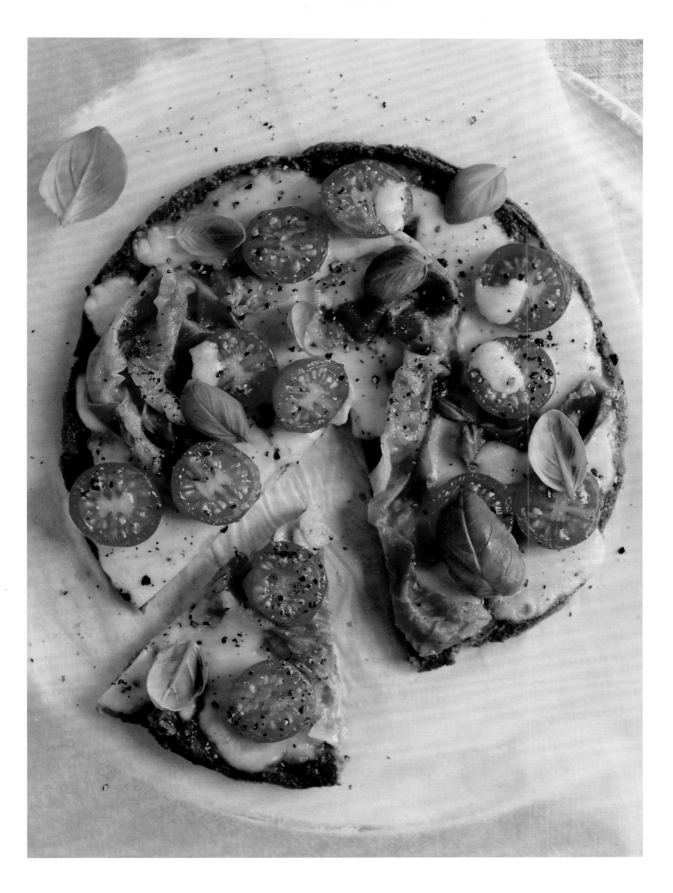

Scotch egg with crunchy nut crust

Shop-bought Scotch eggs frequently have many additives pumped into them, such as extra sugars, stabilisers and trans fats – none of which are good news for anyone. However, with such simple ingredients, a few extra seeds and some spices, these homemade Scotch eggs are delicious, nutritious and protein-packed, without any negative health or blood sugar implications.

They taste amazing straight from the oven with a salad or served cold. With only natural blood sugar-friendly ingredients, this recipe is proof on a plate that everything tastes better when you make it yourself!

 MAKES 3 LARGE SCOTCH EGGS **10 MINS** **15 MINS**

3 large eggs, plus
1 beaten egg

2 tbsp ground almonds
(I use the dried almond
meal left over from my
Almond milk recipe – see
pages 65–6)

1 tsp sea salt and a pinch
of cracked black pepper

100g mixed seeds

6 sausages, skin removed
(100 per cent organic
meat if possible)

1 tsp paprika

1 tsp dried sage

4 tbsp olive oil

To serve

Tomato and sweet paprika
sauce (see page 144)

rocket leaves

Avocado and tomato salsa
(see page 48)

1. Preheat the oven to 200°C/400°F/gas mark 6.

2. Cook the 3 eggs in boiling water for 6 minutes (medium eggs: 5 minutes, small eggs: 4 minutes) then plunge into ice-cold water to stop them cooking. Drain and leave to cool, then peel.

3. Blitz the ground almonds, ½ teaspoon of salt and the mixed seeds in a blender until coarse and crumbly. Tip onto a plate and set aside.

4. Blitz the sausagemeat, paprika and sage, beaten egg, ½ teaspoon salt and a pinch of pepper in the blender until fully combined and sticky.

5. Split the sausage mixture into 3 balls. Using the palm of your hand, create a 'cup' and flatten the ball of sausagemeat into a patty shape in your palm. Place a soft-boiled egg in the middle of the sausagemeat and carefully work the mixture around the egg, making sure you seal and smooth all the sides. Roll the ball in the mixed seeds and almond mixture. Repeat with the remaining 2 eggs.

6. Heat the olive oil over high heat in a frying pan and fry the Scotch eggs, one at a time, for 1–2 minutes until golden all over, then remove using a slotted spoon and place on a baking sheet. When all the eggs have been fried, bake them in the oven for 5–6 minutes. Serve with tomato sauce, rocket leaves and salsa.

NOTE: This recipe makes 3 large Scotch eggs, but you could make 5 smaller ones if you use small eggs.

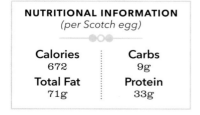

NUTRITIONAL INFORMATION _(per Scotch egg)_	
Calories 672	Carbs 9g
Total Fat 71g	Protein 33g

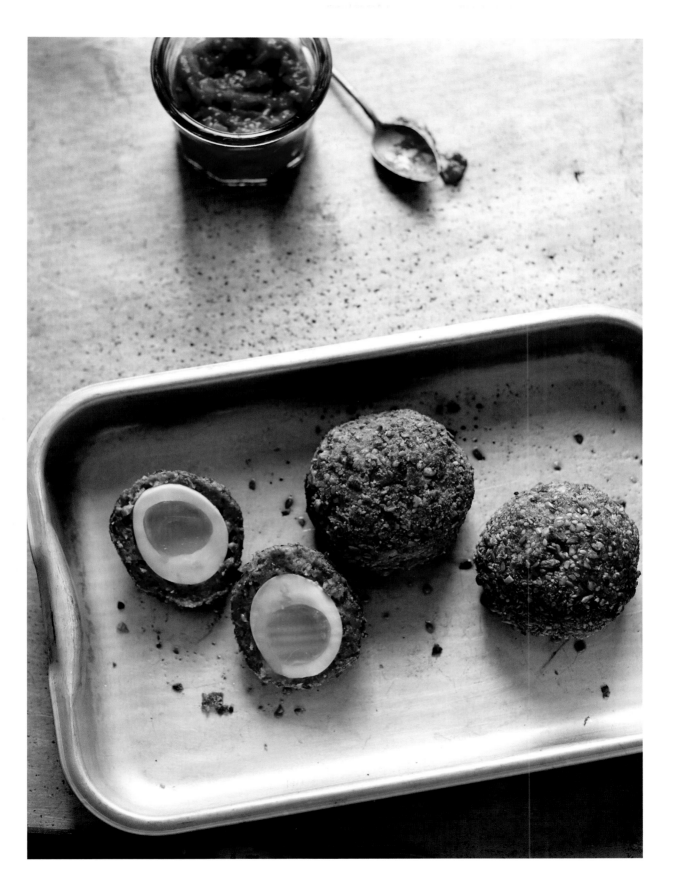

cheese and onion scones

A savoury snack to accompany soup, these scones make the most of one of the most delicious, classic flavour combinations: cheese and onion. They are the perfect replacement to a bread roll; cut them in half and fill them or eat them as they are. They are easy to prepare, and made using only the simplest ingredients.

This recipe makes six medium-sized scones but you could make eight smaller ones or even ten mini ones for a picnic or party. Buttery and moist, with a crunchy outer crust, these are mouthful after mouthful of comforting delight and one recipe that you will want to make again and again!

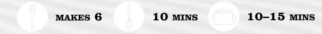

MAKES 6   10 MINS   10–15 MINS

200g ground almonds, plus extra to dust

50g cold butter, cut into smallish cubes, plus extra for greasing

a pinch of sea salt

100g Cheddar cheese, grated

1 spring onion, thinly sliced

1 beaten egg, to glaze

1. Preheat the oven to 200°C/400°F/gas mark 6 and grease a baking sheet.

2. Put the ground almonds, butter and sea salt in a food processor and pulse until the mixture resembles breadcrumbs. If you do not have a food processor you can do this by hand by rubbing the cubes of butter into the ground almonds in a bowl until combined and crumbly.

3. Put the mixture in a large bowl and add the cheese and spring onion. Combine well.

4. Make a well in the centre of the dry ingredients and very slowly pour in 25ml cold water until the dough has come together. It should be slightly sticky.

5. Dust a work surface with some ground almonds and knead the dough together.

6. Dust a rolling pin and roll out the dough to a thickness of 2cm. Cut out scones using a fluted or round cutter of whatever size you prefer, depending on how many scones you wish to make. Gather up the trimmings into a ball, re-roll and cut the remaining dough into rounds. Alternatively, take a squash ball-sized amount of the mixture and mould it into a scone shape.

7. Place the scones on the greased baking sheet and carefully brush the tops with the beaten egg.

8. Bake for 10–15 minutes until golden brown.

9. Transfer to a wire rack and allow to cool before eating. They can be stored in a sealed container for up to 3 days.

NUTRITIONAL INFORMATION
(per serving)

Calories	Carbs
364	8g
Total Fat	Protein
33g	13g

baked cheesy broccoli and spring onion burgers

When you're feeling hungry, but a quick look in the fridge reminds you that you don't have any healthy ready-made dishes, the risk is you will head for the takeaway or convenience store and buy a processed meal, loaded with sugars and carbs. We all do it!

Keep a batch of these burgers in the fridge for a perfect grab-and-go snack. I usually make them on a Sunday and pop them in a Tupperware in the fridge for picking at during the week. The burgers are great for mopping up soups, taking on picnics and as healthy finger food for children's lunchboxes – a perfect substitute for chunks of bread or sandwiches.

 MAKES 9   **10 MINS**   **20 MINS**

300g broccoli, cut into florets and hard stalk removed

50g white onion, cut into quarters

½ tsp each sea salt and cracked black pepper

50g mature Cheddar cheese, grated

50g mozzarella, grated

½ tsp dried sage

2 large eggs, beaten

4 tbsp ground almonds

1 spring onion (15g), finely chopped

1 tbsp olive oil, plus extra for greasing (optional)

1. Preheat the oven to 200°C/400°F/gas mark 6 and grease a baking sheet with oil or line it with greaseproof paper.

2. Put the broccoli and onion in a blender or food processor and pulse to a couscous-like consistency (about 3–4 pulses). Alternatively, grate the broccoli by hand and finely dice the onion with a sharp knife.

3. Put the broccoli and onion mixture, salt and pepper, 25g of the Cheddar, all the mozzarella and sage in a large bowl and combine well.

4. Add the beaten eggs and ground almonds, then the remaining grated Cheddar, the finely chopped spring onion and oil, and combine: the mixture should be thick and not runny.

5. Spoon out a golf ball-sized amount of the mixture and mould it into a burger shape, then place on the baking sheet. Repeat until all the mixture has been used up (you should get 9 burgers from the mixture).

6. Bake for about 20 minutes until nicely browned on top – if you make them bigger or smaller, adjust the cooking time accordingly.

7. Serve these straightaway or transfer them to a wire rack to cool – the longer you can let them cool the firmer they will be and, in my opinion, the tastier! Store in a sealed container in the fridge for up to 3 days.

NUTRITIONAL INFORMATION	
(per burger)	
Calories	Carbs
90	4g
Total Fat	Protein
7g	6g

pea and feta fritters

These fresh, savoury fritters are an incredibly tasty savoury snack or lunchtime accompaniment. They make a great replacement for bread and are delicious dipped into soup.

The pea and feta combination works beautifully – the texture of the fritters is so moreish it feels like they should be loaded with carbs and naughty additives, but the ingredients are simple, packed with goodness and are, of course, blood sugar-friendly.

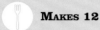 MAKES 12    10 MINS   20 MINS

250g frozen peas
20g coconut flour
60g ground almonds
4 large eggs
2 spring onions (about 30g), thinly sliced
60g crumbled feta
1 tbsp coconut oil
sea salt and cracked black pepper

1. Boil a pan of water over high heat and add the frozen peas. Bring back to the boil then reduce the heat and simmer for about 4 minutes until the peas are tender and cooked. Drain, then run under cold water for a minute until cool.

2. Once the peas are cool, put three-quarters of them into a food processor or blender along with the coconut flour and ground almonds. Blitz until well combined.

3. Add the eggs, spring onions, 30g of the crumbled feta, some salt and pepper and then blitz again until the mixture is well combined and has the consistency of a thick batter. Transfer to a bowl and stir in the remaining crumbled feta.

4. Melt the coconut oil in a non-stick frying pan over high heat.

5. After 1 minute, turn to low heat and add spoonfuls of the batter. Cook for 3–4 minutes until browned on the underside and easy to flip, then flip and cook on the other side for 3–4 minutes until cooked through. You may need to do this in batches.

6. Place the cooked fritters on a wire rack set over some baking parchment.

7. Serve warm or allow to cool and serve cold. Store in a sealed container in the fridge until required.

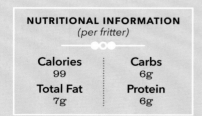

NUTRITIONAL INFORMATION
(per fritter)

Calories	Carbs
99	6g
Total Fat	**Protein**
7g	6g

carrot and coriander fritters

These fritters are very quick and easy to prepare, and perfect as a snack, vegetable side dish or a healthy, filling and colourful lunchbox option for children.

Before cooking the whole batch, cook one fritter to ensure the stiffness of the mixture is correct so that it doesn't collapse in the pan, then make adjustments to the rest of the mixture if necessary (if the mixture is too thick, add an extra egg).

For those of you who enjoy spicy, hot dishes, add some curry powder to taste.

 MAKES 13   **15 MINS** (PLUS OPTIONAL 15 MINS IN THE OVEN REHEATING)   **16–20 MINS**

2 carrots (about 230g)

4 spring onions (about 60g), finely chopped

2 tsp ground coriander

3 tbsp ground almonds

2 large eggs, beaten

4 tbsp olive oil

sea salt and cracked black pepper

1. Coarsely grate the carrots by hand with a box grater and remove any moisture by patting the grated carrot dry with kitchen paper or enclosing it in a clean tea towel and squeezing out the liquid.

2. Put the carrots, spring onions, coriander, ground almonds and some salt and pepper in a large bowl. Mix well to combine, then stir in the beaten eggs.

3. Heat 2 tablespoons of the olive oil in a large non-stick frying pan over medium-high heat. When the oil is hot, try cooking 1 fritter. Add 1 heaped tablespoon of the mixture to the pan and flatten it. Be careful – the oil may spit. Fry for about 2 minutes then flip and fry for a further 2–3 minutes until golden brown. If you are unable to flip the fritter, cook it for a little longer before trying again.

4. Place the cooked fritter on a wire rack set over some baking parchment to cool. Repeat, adding extra oil to the pan as needed, until all the mixture has been used up. I usually make 2–3 fritters in the pan at a time.

5. Once you have cooked them all, dab off any extra oil with kitchen paper. Cool and enjoy later.

6. If you want to serve them hot, pop on a baking sheet in the oven at 170°C/325°F/gas mark 3 for 15 minutes. Serve immediately.

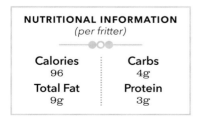

NUTRITIONAL INFORMATION
(per fritter)

Calories	Carbs
96	4g
Total Fat	**Protein**
9g	3g

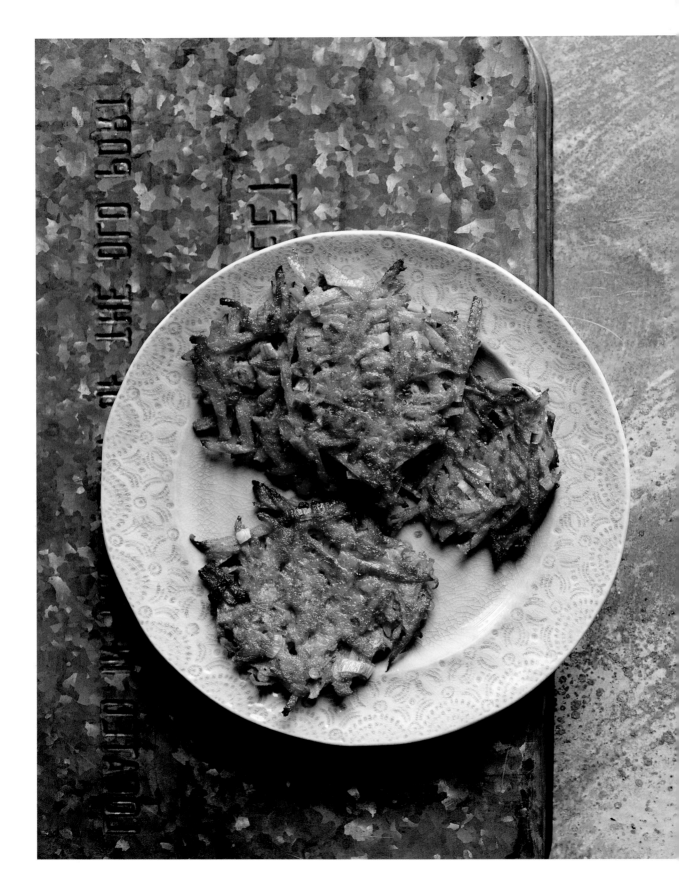

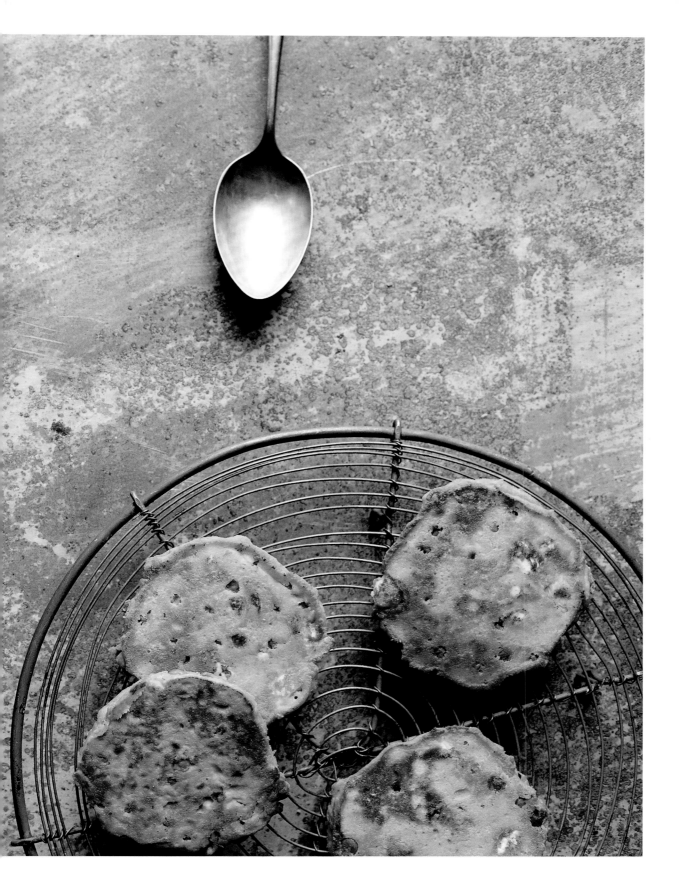

red pepper and Brazil nut mushrooms

Here's a delicious, simple and nutrient-packed dish that can be enjoyed for breakfast, lunch or dinner. The red pepper works beautifully with the Brazil nuts, almonds and coriander to give a crunchy, flavour-filled topping to the meaty mushrooms. If you want to reduce the carb content, swap the red pepper for a green or yellow one, or perhaps use spinach or broccoli in its place. Add some baked salmon or a fried egg for extra protein.

 4   **15 MINS**   **35 MINS**

100g red pepper, deseeded and cut into large chunks

50g Brazil nuts

50g almonds

a small handful of coriander (12–14 leaves)

½ tsp sea salt

150g Portobello mushrooms (about 4 large mushrooms)

1. Preheat the oven to 200°C/400°F/gas mark 6.

2. Bake the red pepper chunks on a baking tray for 15 minutes until soft and slightly browned. Leave the oven on.

3. Put the red pepper, Brazil nuts, almonds, coriander and salt in a food processor or blender and blitz for 1–2 minutes until fully combined and a chunky paste-like consistency.

4. Cut the stalks out of the mushrooms so that there's a well in which to place the red pepper mixture.

5. Place the mushrooms on a baking sheet and fill each with 1 tablespoon of the red pepper mixture, flattening it out a little.

6. Cook in the oven for about 20 minutes, until the mushrooms are cooked through and the red pepper mix has toasted on top. Serve straightaway.

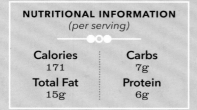

NUTRITIONAL INFORMATION
(per serving)

Calories	Carbs
171	7g
Total Fat	**Protein**
15g	6g

pesto muffins

Every time I make these muffins I do so with the intention of having them in the fridge for the week, so that if anyone's hungry there is something delicious to hand. However, no sooner are they made, than they are eaten – they are even a favourite with my friend's children. The pesto adds another dimension to the egg, but add as much or as little garlic to it as you want (I realise that garlic at lunchtime, especially if you are working in close proximity to others, may well be a no!).

These muffins are easy to transport in a lunchbox and are perfect for a low-carb picnic treat: they are virtually carb free.

 MAKES 6   **15 MINS**   **20–25 MINS**

100g unsalted cashew nuts

50g basil leaves

40g spinach leaves

1 garlic clove, peeled (optional)

80ml olive oil, plus extra for greasing (if needed)

6 large eggs

sea salt and cracked black pepper

1. Preheat the oven to 200°C/400°F/gas mark 6 and grease 6 holes in a muffin tin or fill with paper cases. (I prefer to use a silicone cupcake/muffin mould as they are non-stick, making it easier to remove the baked muffins.)

2. First, make the pesto. Blitz the cashew nuts, basil, spinach, garlic (if using), ½ teaspoon of salt and a generous pinch of pepper in a blender or food processor to a coarse paste. On low speed, pour in the olive oil a little at a time until a paste has formed (have a taste, and add more salt if you like). You will probably have to use a spatula to scrape down the sides. Set aside.

3. Now, make the muffins. Whisk the eggs with 2 tablespoons of water and a pinch of salt and pepper.

4. Pour the egg mix equally into the 6 muffin holes or cases so that they are three-quarters full.

5. Spoon 1 teaspoon of the pesto mix into each individual egg cup. Bake in the oven for 20–25 minutes until well risen, golden and fully set.

6. Remove from the oven and allow to cool in the tin for 5–10 minutes, then serve immediately or leave on a wire rack to cool fully before placing in a sealed container in the fridge for up to 5 days.

NUTRITIONAL INFORMATION
(per muffin)

Calories	Carbs
274	7g
Total Fat	**Protein**
25g	10g

picnic rolls

These are a great substitute for bread rolls and are incredibly simple to make. They are very low in carbs, protein-packed and filling. One long roll serves two people, but you can cut it into small finger-food rolls or have them a little thicker. They can be filled with whatever you desire, and are great for taking to work for lunch to have alongside some Sea salt and lemon zest almonds (see page 186). My Avocado and chilli cream dip recipe (see page 125) also makes for a delicious spread, as well as some fresh and flavourful ingredients such as cooked ham, sliced tomato and cucumber. (See below for more filling options.)

 2   **5 MINS**   **16 MINS, PLUS COOLING**

butter or oil, for greasing

4 large eggs

3 tbsp mixed seeds

a handful of spinach leaves, finely chopped

12 basil leaves, finely chopped

a pinch each of sea salt and cracked black pepper

1. Preheat the oven to 200°C/400°F/gas mark 6 and line a greased baking tray with greaseproof paper.

2. Crack the eggs into a mixing bowl and whisk. Set aside.

3. Dry-toast the mixed seeds in a frying pan for a minute or two until golden brown. Add the seeds and the chopped leaves to the egg, season and combine well.

4. Pour the mixture over the greaseproof paper on the baking tray and spread out evenly. Bake for about 15 minutes until golden brown and cooked through.

5. Lift the ends of the greaseproof paper and flip the cooked mixture onto a wire rack to cool.

6. Place your chosen filling ingredients (see below) horizontally along the length of the egg base in lines, from one side to the other, then roll from the long side and, using a sharp knife, cut into bite-sized rolls. Serve with other finger food or salad, or immediately wrap in cling film and place in the fridge until required.

FILLING OPTIONS:

- 2 slices goat's cheese, 1 sliced fig and a handful of rocket
- 1 mashed avocado, 3 medium mushrooms, sliced and fried, a pinch of sea salt

- 1 tbsp full-fat cream cheese, 1 thin strip of smoked salmon and 2 chives, finely chopped
- 4 sliced cherry tomatoes, ¼ sliced small red onion, 100g cooked chicken strips

---

NUTRITIONAL INFORMATION
(per unfilled roll)

Calories	Carbs
269	8g
Total Fat	**Protein**
19g	20g

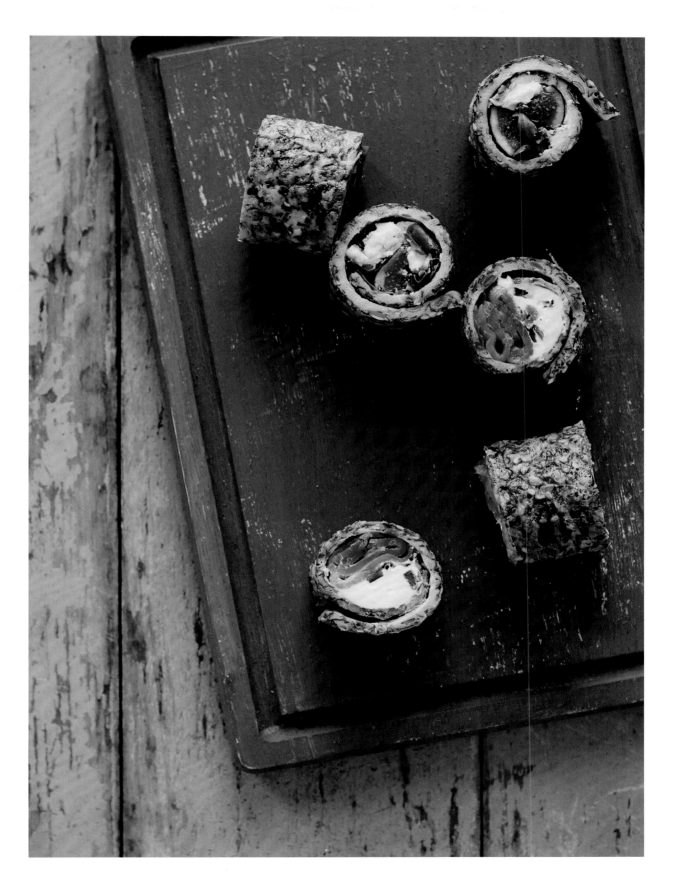

cauliflower and cashew dip

Think hummus, but without any blood sugar-raising chickpeas. Packed with fresh and delicious flavours, this is a dip for the whole family to have with salad or with crackers (see page 187), to slather on a slice of bread (see page 198), or as a side to my Brilliant beef burgers (see page 151). This is certainly one of the lowest-carb dips you will find, but it's also thick, creamy and incredibly moreish.

Make sure you soak the cashews for at least three hours before using them, as this will ensure the creamiest consistency possible.

 6   **10 MINS, PLUS 3 HOURS SOAKING**   **15 MINS**

100g unsalted cashew nuts

115g cauliflower, cut into florets, tough stalks removed

1 garlic clove, peeled

juice of ½ lemon

3 tbsp coconut milk or other nut milk

sea salt and cracked black pepper

1. Put the cashew nuts in a bowl, cover with water and leave to soak for at least 3 hours.

2. While the nuts are soaking, add the cauliflower florets to a small pan of water, bring to the boil and cook for around 15 minutes until soft and tender. Drain and set aside to cool.

3. Drain the cashew nuts and place them in a food processor or blender. Blitz on high speed with the garlic clove, cooked cauliflower, lemon juice and coconut milk until smooth, thick and creamy.

4. Season with salt and pepper to taste, and serve.

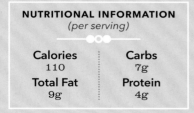

NUTRITIONAL INFORMATION
(per serving)

Calories	Carbs
110	7g
Total Fat	**Protein**
9g	4g

roasted butternut squash and lemony yoghurt dip

The whole family can enjoy this healthy, homemade dip. It is blood sugar-friendly, light and fresh and incredibly simple to make. Perfect for serving with a salad, with homemade fish or vegetable skewers or as a dip to share with some crudités, or spread over my Super seed bread (see page 198).

The butternut squash is subtly sweet and works beautifully with the tartness of the lemon. Crack some black pepper on top for added heat.

 4 **10** MINS **45** MINS

280g butternut squash, peeled, deseeded and cut into 2.5cm chunks

1 tbsp olive oil

100g full-fat plain yoghurt

grated zest of ½ lemon, plus extra to garnish

sea salt and cracked black pepper

1. Preheat the oven to 200°C/400°F/gas mark 6.

2. Put the butternut squash chunks on a baking tray, then sprinkle with some sea salt and black pepper, drizzle with the olive oil and bake for about 45 minutes until it is soft and the edges are browned.

3. Roughly mash the squash chunks or place them in a blender or food processor with the yoghurt and lemon zest and blitz until smooth and creamy.

4. Spoon the dip into a dish, garnish it with an extra grating of lemon zest and serve with whatever accompaniments you fancy.

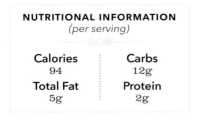

NUTRITIONAL INFORMATION
(per serving)

Calories	Carbs
94	12g
Total Fat	**Protein**
5g	2g

homemade mayonnaise

This recipe for mayonnaise makes a great alternative to shop-bought mayonnaise, which is typically high in carbohydrates and has added sugars and starch. Cubes of fried chorizo or fresh feta make scrumptious additions, too.

 6 5 MINS

250ml light olive oil or avocado oil

1 large egg, room temperature

1 tbsp apple cider vinegar

juice of ½ lemon

½ tsp salt and ½ tsp cracked black pepper (optional)

1. Put the oil in a deep jug or bowl, then crack in the egg and add the rest of the ingredients.

2. If you are using a hand-held blender, place the blender at the bottom of the bowl and blitz – it will immediately thicken and turn into a mayonnaise colour and consistency. I would blend for at least 1 minute to ensure a very smooth and creamy texture.

3. Have a taste test and add extra salt or lemon juice, if you like.

4. Spoon into a jar, seal and keep in the fridge for up to 14 days.

NOTE: Ideally use a hand-held blender to make this mayonnaise. You can whisk by hand, but it will take a little longer and requires a lot of elbow grease.

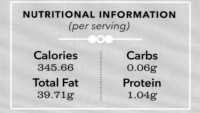

NUTRITIONAL INFORMATION
(per serving)

Calories	Carbs
345.66	0.06g
Total Fat	**Protein**
39.71g	1.04g

avocado and chilli cream dip

This is really simple to make, fresh and flavourful, with blood sugar-friendly ingredients. It's perfect for serving with a salad, as a dip with some crudités, with roasted vegetables or on the side of my Sesame chicken goujons (see page 138) or Coconut chicken nuggets (see page 144).

 4 **5 MINS**

1 large ripe avocado, halved, de-stoned and peeled

75ml coconut milk or your favourite milk, such as almond

½ red chilli, deseeded and finely chopped, plus extra to garnish

juice of ½ small lime

sea salt and cracked black pepper

1. Blitz the avocado flesh in a blender or food processor, or mash it by hand in a bowl.

2. Add the coconut milk, chilli, lime juice and a pinch of salt and blitz or mash until creamy.

3. Transfer to a pretty serving bowl and decorate with some finely diced chilli.

NOTE: To change up the dip, you could top it with toasted seeds, toasted coconut flakes or finely chopped spring onion.

NUTRITIONAL INFORMATION	
(per serving)	
Calories 116	**Carbs** 5.49g
Total Fat 10.71g	**Protein** 1.34g

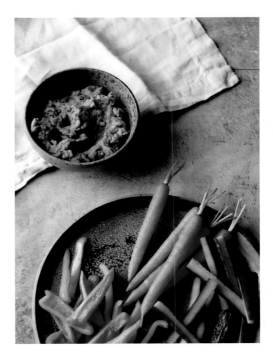

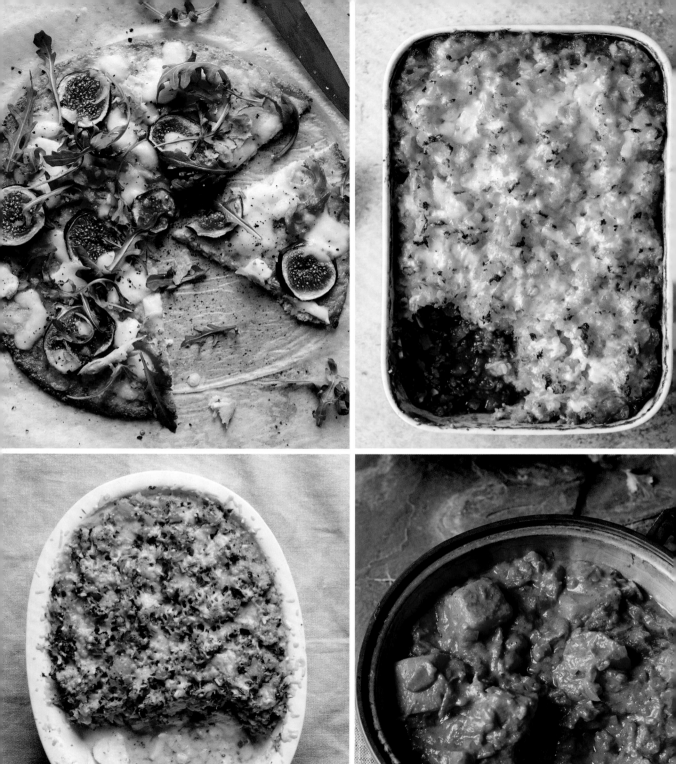

Dinners

How to ROAST A CHICKEN

Everyone has their own method when it comes to roasting a chicken; some are more complicated than others, but this is my favourite method.

Chicken is a delicious meat – lean and relatively inexpensive, it can be partnered with many different flavours, spices and accompaniments or enjoyed simply on its own. It can be grilled, fried, barbecued, baked, roasted, grilled – you name it!

Where possible, always opt for organic and free-range chicken as it is undoubtedly tastier. You may well have to pay a little more, but it is the best option, especially when it comes to the welfare of the bird and sustainability.

One of the great things about roasting a chicken is the leftovers. If there are only a couple of you, buying a bigger bird to roast can end up being quite economical, as it provides you with at least three speedy meals in the days after you've enjoyed the roast, such as fajitas (see page 140), salads or curries.

Remove the chicken from the fridge 30 minutes before roasting and let it sit at room temperature.

 8　 **10 MINS**　 **APPROX. 2 HOURS 10 MINS**

1 tbsp olive oil, plus extra for drizzling

3 red onions (about 360g), peeled, stalk and root removed, then cut into chunks widthways

6 whole garlic cloves, peeled

1 large chicken (approximately 2.35kg)

sea salt and cracked black pepper

1. Preheat the oven to 210°C/420°F/gas mark 7.

2. Drizzle the tablespoon of olive oil onto a large roasting tray and arrange the red onion chunks cut-side down. Scatter in the garlic cloves – you want the chicken to cover them. Place the chicken on top of the onion and garlic, generously drizzle with olive oil and season well all over with salt and pepper.

3. Place the roasting tray in the middle of the oven and cook for 1 hour 30 minutes, reducing the heat to 140°C/280°F/gas mark 1 for the final 30–40 minutes. If there are a lot of cooking juices in the roasting tray, spoon them over the chicken to create a crispier skin.

4. Use a meat thermometer to check that the centre of the bird has cooked through or pierce the thigh with a knife to see if the juices run clear. If there are any traces of blood in the juice, return the chicken to the oven until cooked.

5. Remove from the oven, cover the chicken with foil and leave it to rest for 10–15 minutes before serving.

NOTE: Strip the carcass of any leftover meat and keep in the fridge, covered, for up to 2 days.

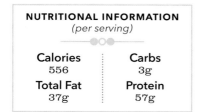

NUTRITIONAL INFORMATION
(per serving)

Calories	Carbs
556	3g
Total Fat	**Protein**
37g	57g

chicken stock

If you have roasted a free-range or organic chicken you can boil the carcass to make a stock (the better the quality of the chicken, the more pleasant the flavour, and the more nutritional benefits you will get from the stock). The great thing about homemade stock is that you control exactly what goes in to it, safe in the knowledge that you aren't consuming unnecessary added salts and sugars.

Stocks are the foundation of many important and delicious kitchen creations and are so easy to make.

 Makes about 3 litres   **15 mins**   **6 hours 15 mins**

1 whole chicken carcass

500g washed and roughly chopped mixed vegetables, such as carrots, onion, leek and celery

bouquet garni made of coriander, basil, thyme, flat-leaf parsley, bay leaf (see Note)

1 tsp sea salt

5 black peppercorns

1. Chop up the carcass to fit the bones into a large casserole or stock pot, making sure you have stripped off all the meat – keep that to use in another dish.

2. Place the bones in the pot over high heat, cover with about 4.5 litres of cold water, bring to the boil and boil for 10–15 minutes, then turn down to a simmer. Use a large spoon to skim off any scum from the top of the water.

3. Add the vegetables, bouquet garni, salt and peppercorns and simmer for about 6 hours, skimming the surface every now and then.

4. Strain the stock through a fine sieve and pour the stock into jam jars or other containers to use when needed. Seal and store in the fridge for up to 4 or 5 days or freeze until required.

Note: You can make a bouquet garni with a small piece of muslin and a hair band or length of kitchen string. Place all the herbs in the centre of the muslin (I like to use 1 tbsp dried flat-leaf parsley, 1 tsp dried basil, 1 tsp dried thyme and 1 bay leaf,) gather up the sides and tie the hair band or string around it to seal it and stop the herbs escaping.

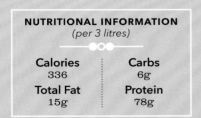

NUTRITIONAL INFORMATION
(per 3 litres)

Calories	Carbs
336	6g
Total Fat	**Protein**
15g	78g

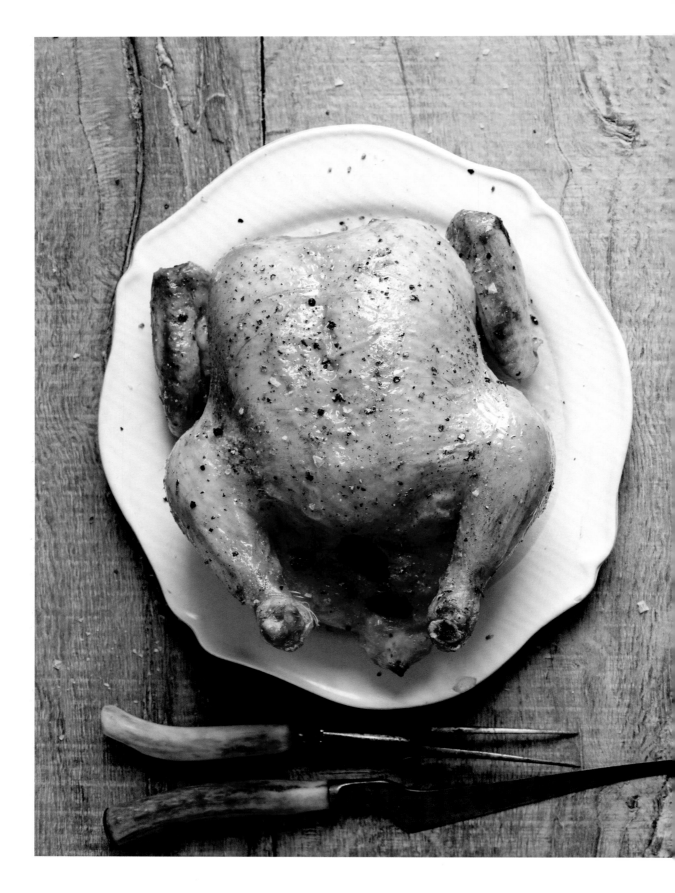

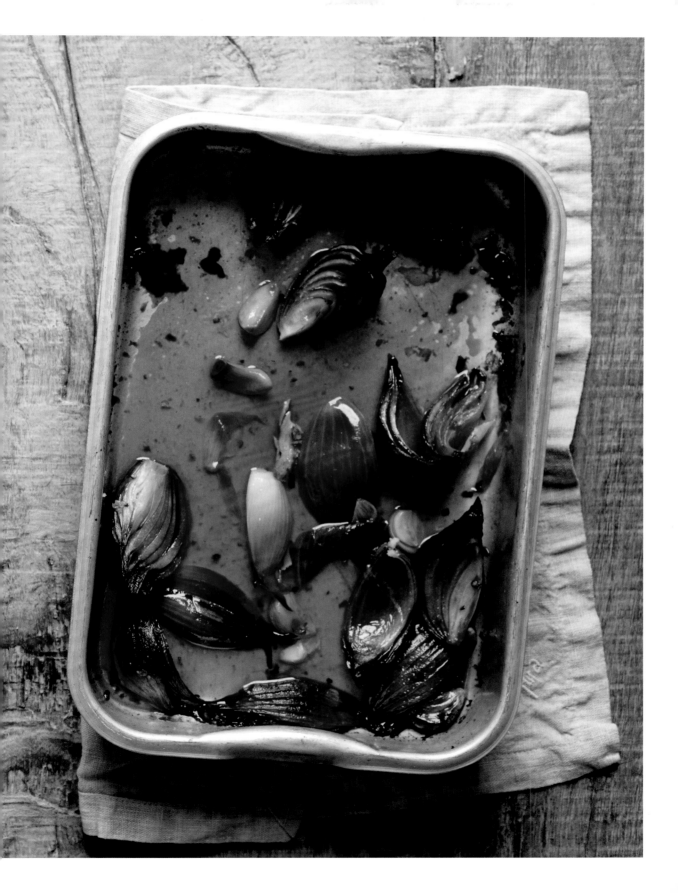

coconut chicken tikka

This rich, thick and aromatic curry is made with coconut cream and lots of delicious spices. Herbs and spices are amazing: they are full of so many healing, antibacterial and antiviral properties and some also contain more disease-fighting antioxidants than fruits and vegetables. The best thing about them is that they have no nasty additives or extra sugars so you can create vibrant, authentic dishes without worrying about pumping your body full of sugars and stabilisers.

This is my version of the classic chicken tikka curry, made with only blood sugar-friendly ingredients, and I can safely say that this is one of my favourite recipes. It is perfect comfort food.

 4   10 MINS   40 MINS

1 tsp coconut oil

3 garlic cloves, crushed

1 medium white onion (about 225g), finely chopped

2 tsp Tikka spice mix (see page 106)

350g skinless and boneless chicken thighs, chopped into bite-sized pieces

1 x 400g tin chopped tomatoes

230ml coconut cream (scooped off the top of a chilled 400ml tin of full-fat coconut milk – see Note)

Coconut cauliflower rice (see recipe opposite), to serve

coriander leaves, to garnish

1. Melt the coconut oil in a large pan over high heat. Add the garlic and onion and fry for 2–3 minutes until softened and turning golden brown. Add the spice mix and fry for a further 2–3 minutes. If the ingredients start to stick, stir in 2–3 tablespoons of water, a little at a time.

2. Add the chopped chicken and coat it with the tikka-onion mixture. Fry for 3–4 minutes, then add the chopped tomatoes plus 500ml water and reduce the heat to low so the liquid is just simmering. Cook for at least 25 minutes until the sauce has reduced.

3. Stir in the coconut cream and cook for a further 2–3 minutes before serving.

4. Serve with coconut cauliflower rice, garnished with coriander leaves.

NOTES: Bear in mind, if serving the curry with the cauliflower rice opposite, that a single serving of cauliflower rice contains 89 calories, 4g fat, 11g carbs and 4g protein.

You can buy coconut cream or prepare it yourself by popping a tin of coconut milk in the fridge for a minimum of 5 hours. The liquid will separate from the cream, so when you open the tin you can scoop the cream off the top. If there isn't enough cream, add a little of the liquid beneath until you have what you need.

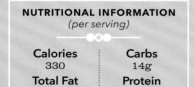

NUTRITIONAL INFORMATION
(per serving)

Calories	Carbs
330	14g
Total Fat	**Protein**
18g	29g

almond butter chicken curry

This is one of the creamiest and most indulgent curries I have ever made. It tastes like it has been cooking for hours, but the truth is it takes just 35 minutes to make. It's living proof that cooking doesn't have to be over-complicated. It can be enjoyed straightaway or made in advance and reheated. The longer the flavours have to infuse, the better.

The cauliflower rice, one of the best and most satisfying rice alternatives, ensures your blood sugar remains stable during and after the meal.

 4   **10 MINS**   **25 MINS**

For the curry

2 tsp coconut oil

1 large white onion (about 340g), finely chopped

2 garlic cloves, finely chopped

460g skinless and boneless chicken breast, cut into bite-sized chunks

1 tsp ground cumin

2 tsp curry powder

½ tsp sea salt

2 tbsp smooth almond butter or other nut butter

For the coconut cauliflower rice

1 large cauliflower (750g), cut into florets, tough stalks removed

3 tbsp desiccated coconut

1 tsp sea salt

1 tsp ground turmeric

2 tsp coconut oil

1. Melt the coconut oil in a deep wok over high heat, then add the onion and garlic and fry for 3–4 minutes until lightly browned and soft. Add the chicken and fry until cooked through, then reduce the heat to medium and add the spices and salt, coating the chicken in the mixture. Fry for another 1–2 minutes until fragrant. Mix in 1 tablespoon of water, then reduce the heat to low and add the nut butter along with 250ml water. Gently stir all the ingredients together until a creamy sauce has formed, then simmer for 10–15 minutes (the mixture will thicken considerably during this time). If it thickens too much add 1–2 tablespoons of water at a time until you reach the desired consistency.

2. Meanwhile, make the coconut cauliflower rice. Blitz the cauliflower florets in a food processor until they have a rice-like consistency. Alternatively, use a box grater to grate the cauliflower by hand. Put the grated cauliflower in a piece of muslin, or a sieve lined with kitchen paper set over a bowl, and allow all the water to drain away. Once drained, pop the rice into a large dish, and mix in the desiccated coconut, salt and turmeric.

3. Melt the coconut oil in a deep wok or pan over high heat. Carefully add the cauliflower rice and cook for 5 minutes, stirring it regularly so that it does not stick. The rice should still be grainy and should still retain a bite.

4. Serve the curry with the warm coconut cauliflower rice.

NUTRITIONAL INFORMATION
(per serving)

Calories	Carbs
422	23g
Total Fat	**Protein**
21g	41g

creamy cashew chicken with tarragon and lemon

This is an incredibly simple dish to make; light, filling and flavour-packed, with protein, good fats and, most importantly, low in carbs. The cashew cream needs to be made in advance so that the cashews are soft enough to give the curry its delicious creamy texture.

 The perfect alternative to a takeaway, or excellent served up on an evening in or at an informal dinner party dish, I like to serve this alongside a bed of wilted spinach and some steamed Tenderstem broccoli, but if you are looking for something a little more substantial, you could try my Coconut cauliflower rice (see page 133 and nutritional data on page 132).

 4   **10 MINS, PLUS 40 MINS SOAKING TIME**   **20 MINS**

130g unsalted cashew nuts

115g full-fat Greek yoghurt

1 tsp sea salt, plus extra to taste

1 tbsp olive oil

3 garlic cloves, thinly sliced

600g skinless, boneless chicken breast, diced

3 tsp dried tarragon

1 lemon, for squeezing

cracked black pepper

1. First, make the cashew cream. Pop the cashew nuts into a bowl and cover with cold water, then leave to soak for 40 minutes.

2. Drain the cashew nuts, discarding the soaking water, and put the nuts into a blender or food processor with the Greek yoghurt, sea salt and 100ml of water. Blitz until the mixture has a creamy consistency.

3. Heat the olive oil in a wok or large pan over high heat, add the garlic cloves and fry for 30–40 seconds, then add the chicken and fry for about 4 minutes until lightly browned and cooked through.

4. Add the dried tarragon, the cashew cream and another 100ml water and bring to the boil, then reduce the heat to low and simmer for 15 minutes, stirring every so often, until the sauce has thickened.

5. Add salt and pepper to taste and a generous squeeze of lemon at the end, stir and serve.

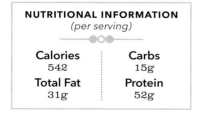

NUTRITIONAL INFORMATION
(per serving)

Calories	Carbs
542	15g
Total Fat	**Protein**
31g	52g

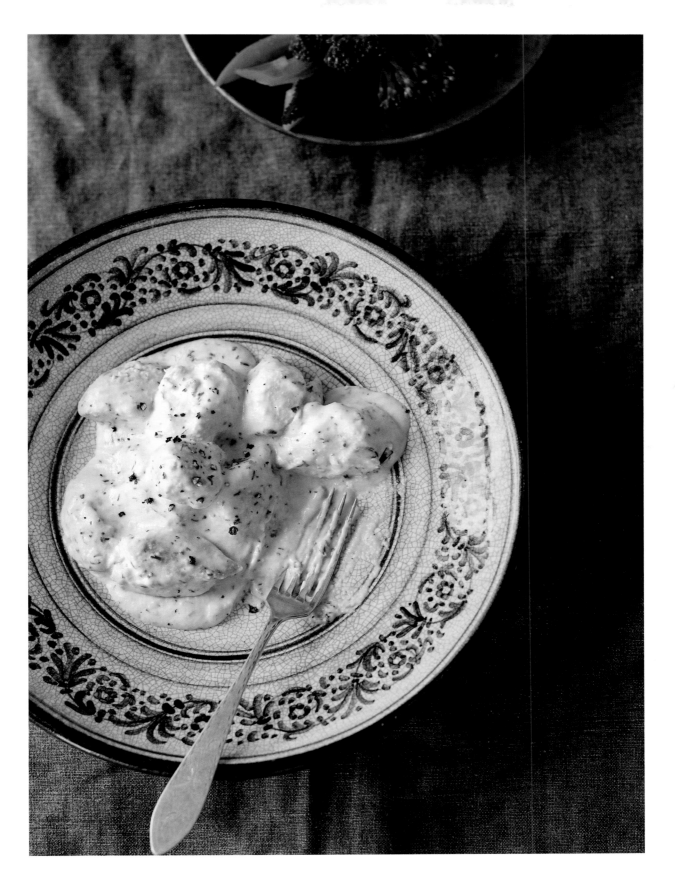

egg-fried cauliflower rice with chicken

This recipe is a classic twist on a favourite takeaway dish. Perfect for feeding the whole family quickly, it definitely tastes too good to be true but is free of additives, blood sugar-inducing grains and excessive salt. It's got the same taste and texture as the takeaway version and is incredibly easy to make.

 4   10 MINS   20 MINS

400g cauliflower, cut into florets and tough stalks removed

1 tbsp coconut oil

530g skinless and boneless chicken thighs, diced

1 tbsp smoked paprika

1 tbsp ground coriander

1 tsp ground cumin

170g red pepper, deseeded and thinly sliced

1 garlic clove, thinly sliced

150g red onion, diced

½ red chilli, deseeded and chopped

½ piece fresh root ginger, grated

300ml vegetable stock

1 tbsp sesame oil or olive oil

juice of ½ lemon

2 eggs, whisked

2 spring onions, shredded, to garnish

coriander leaves, to garnish

1. Start by making the cauliflower rice. Blitz the cauliflower florets in a food processor until they have a rice-like consistency. Alternatively, use a box grater to grate the cauliflower by hand. Put the grated cauliflower in a piece of muslin, or a sieve lined with kitchen paper set over a bowl and allow all the water to drain away.

2. While the cauliflower rice drains, melt the coconut oil in a wok or heavy frying pan over medium heat, then add the chicken and fry for 2–3 minutes until cooked through.

3. Add half the spices to the chicken and fry for 3–4 minutes until golden and fragrant, then add the pepper, garlic, onion, chilli and ginger to the chicken and continue to fry for 3–4 minutes until the vegetables have softened.

4. Add half the vegetable stock to the pan, reduce the heat to low and cook for 2–3 minutes to thicken the liquid slightly.

5. Once the stock has reduced, add the cauliflower rice to the pan with the remaining spices. Continue to cook, stirring, for 2–3 minutes.

6. Add the remaining stock and simmer for a further 5 minutes. Once the stock has reduced, add the sesame or olive oil, lemon juice and the whisked eggs. Cook for 30 seconds then stir thoroughly and serve straightaway, garnished with shredded spring onions and coriander.

NUTRITIONAL INFORMATION
(per serving)

Calories	Carbs
412	19g
Total Fat	**Protein**
17g	47g

pesto baked chicken

A mouthwatering baked chicken recipe that's simple to make and wonderful served hot or cold with salad or roasted vegetables. The recipe serves four people easily – or two people over two meals. We usually enjoy our second meal cold (when the flavours have had time to infuse, it is even more delicious) on a couple of pieces of homemade bread (see page 198) with sun-dried tomatoes and maybe a little fried halloumi.

I add spinach to pesto to bulk it out and give it an extra dose of iron. Spinach is loaded with goodness, is low in fat, carbs and cholesterol and is packed with all the key vitamins and minerals.

 4   **15 MINS**   **40–45 MINS**

100g spinach leaves

2 handfuls of basil leaves

75g shelled pistachios

2 garlic cloves, peeled

1 tsp sea salt

150ml extra-virgin olive oil

500g skinless and boneless
chicken breasts or thighs

NOTE: You can use any nut here, although pistachios are wonderful and creamy and work incredibly well.

1. Preheat the oven to 220°C/425°F/gas mark 7.

2. First, make the pesto. Put the spinach, basil, pistachios, garlic and salt in a food processor and pulse a few times to roughly combine, then gradually pour in the olive oil while blending, until the mixture is thick and creamy. If it's too thick for your liking, add a little more oil. You will probably have to use a spatula to scrape down the sides.

3. Cut the chicken into strips lengthways (or leave them whole).

4. Spread 1–2 tablespoons of the pesto over the bottom of a non-stick or oiled baking dish, then place the strips of chicken or the whole breasts or thighs carefully on top, packing them next to each other nice and tight. Cover the chicken with the remaining pesto.

5. Place a sheet of foil carefully over the dish, pop it in the oven and bake for 20 minutes.

6. After 20 minutes, reduce the heat to 180°C/350°F/gas mark 4, take the foil off the dish and bake uncovered for a further 20–25 minutes until the top is slightly browned, crisp and the chicken is cooked through (cut a piece of chicken to check the centre is white before serving).

7. Serve straightaway or allow to fully cool before popping in the fridge and enjoying cold. It will keep in the fridge for up to 2 days, in a sealed container.

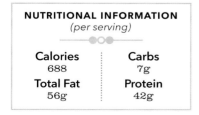

NUTRITIONAL INFORMATION	
(per serving)	
Calories	Carbs
688	7g
Total Fat	Protein
56g	42g

sesame chicken goujons

These 'no nasties' chicken goujons tick all the boxes: fresh, flavoursome, sugar free, dairy free, gluten free, grain free, full of protein and high in vitamins, they are, quite simply, delicious. They are great for kids because there are no additives and they are well and truly p.a.c.k.e.d to the brim with goodness. Be warned, you will definitely be fighting for the last goujon!

 4   15 MINS   10 MINS

2 egg whites

350g skinless and boneless chicken thighs or chicken cut into goujon fillets

75g sesame seeds

1 tsp sea salt

½ tsp cracked black pepper

2-3 tbsp coconut oil or 5-6 tbsp olive oil

To serve

spinach leaves

cherry tomatoes

chopped spring onions

Avocado and chilli cream dip (see page 125)

lime wedges (optional)

1. Using a fork or whisk, beat the egg whites in a shallow bowl until very foamy and beginning to form very slight soft peaks. Set aside.

2. Cut the chicken thighs (if not using ready-prepared goujon fillets) into bite-sized lengths and set aside.

3. Tip the sesame seeds and salt and pepper onto a flat surface and combine and spread out ready for coating your chicken. Set the egg white mix, sesame seeds and chicken in front of you, then take a chicken strip and dip it into the egg white mix first, making sure it's well coated, then roll it in the sesame seeds until fully coated.

4. Repeat with all the chicken pieces (if your egg mix gets a bit 'watery', just whisk it up again until frothy).

5. Heat the oil in a deep frying pan over high heat. When hot, lower the chicken goujons into the oil – being careful as the oil might spit. Cook the chicken goujons for 3–4 minutes on each side until golden.

6. Test one chicken goujon by cutting it in half to make sure they are fully cooked through – the flesh should be white, with no raw pink bits – if not, turn the heat down and continue to cook until done.

7. Serve straightaway with spinach leaves, cherry tomatoes, spring onions, Avocado and chilli cream for dipping and lime wedges for squeezing over, if you like.

NUTRITIONAL INFORMATION (per serving)	
Calories 335	**Carbs** 12g
Total Fat 30g	**Protein** 30g

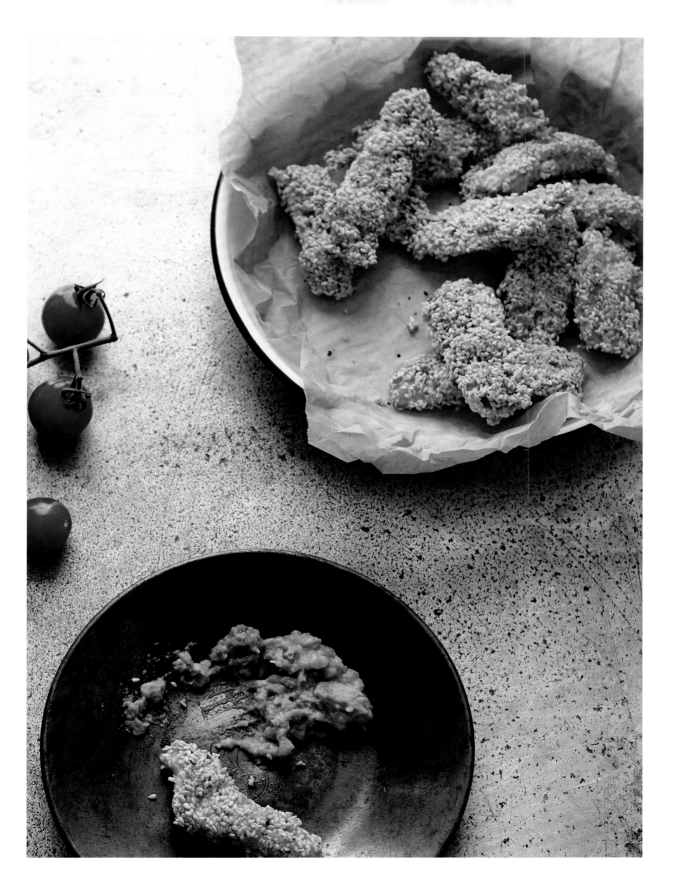

low-carb Mexican style fajitas

This is a great recipe for using up the leftovers from a roast chicken (see page 128). The filling tastes amazing the day you eat it but even better the following day, as the flavours infuse beautifully – you can also serve it on its own with cauliflower rice (see page 133 and nutritional note on page 132). If you do not have any leftover chicken and to save time cooking a chicken, use shop-bought rotisserie chicken for all the deliciousness without the hassle. The divine spice mix can be stored in a small labelled spice jar in the cupboard to use at any time as a dry rub or marinade: it works best on chicken, beef, cod and prawns.

I always make the fajitas first when making this recipe, then leave them cooling on a wire rack, separating each one with kitchen paper. It's hard to believe but the fajitas contain virtually no carbs at all. They are doughy, filling and can be easily rolled to hold whatever you pack into them.

 MAKES 4 TORTILLAS (TO SERVE 2)   **15 MINS**   **15 MINS**

For the tortillas

2 large eggs

40ml coconut milk

2 tsp olive oil

15g coconut flour

½ tsp each sea salt and cracked black pepper

For the fajita spice mix

½ tsp cayenne pepper

1 tsp sea salt

1 tbsp ground cumin

1 tbsp ground coriander

1 tbsp smoked paprika

1 tsp garlic powder

½ tsp cracked black pepper

continues...

1. Preheat the oven to 170°C/325°F/gas mark 3.

2. First, make the tortillas. Whisk together the eggs and coconut milk in a bowl until well combined and frothy, then add the olive oil, coconut flour, and salt and pepper. Whisk together well to make a batter-like consistency.

3. Put a non-stick frying pan over high heat. (If you don't have a non-stick frying pan, coat the bottom of the pan with olive oil before adding the batter.) Add 3 tablespoons of the batter to the centre of the pan and, using the back of a metal spoon, flatten it out into a round tortilla shape. If you accidentally make a hole in the mixture, just fill it in with a little more batter. Reduce the heat to low-medium and cook for about 1 minute until you can slide a spatula under the tortilla and flip it over. The bottom should be lightly browned. If you cannot get the spatula under the sides then give it another 30 seconds before trying again. If the mixture

For the chicken filling
(makes enough for
4 fajitas)

1 tbsp olive oil

1 large white onion (about 340g), thinly sliced

100g red pepper, deseeded and thinly sliced

280g leftover roast chicken (see page 128), cut into bite-sized strips

To serve

1 tbsp per serving grated mature Cheddar cheese

½ avocado, sliced

1 tbsp per serving of homemade Avocado and tomato salsa (see page 48)

1 tbsp per serving soured cream

sticks to the bottom of the pan, make sure the heat is not too high – this will cook the batter too quickly and burn the bottom.

4. Cook the other side for about 1 minute, then remove the tortilla with a spatula and place on a wire rack. Put a piece of greaseproof paper on top and lay the next tortilla on top. Repeat until you have used all the mixture and you have all the tortillas ready to serve.

5. Next, make the fajita spice mix. Put all ingredients in a clean, dry jar. Screw the lid on tightly and shake to combine.

6. Now, make the fajita filling. Heat half the olive oil in a shallow frying pan or wok and fry the onion and pepper for 1 minute. Add 1 teaspoon of the fajita spice mix and fry for 1–1½ minutes until the onion and pepper are soft, then add the remaining oil and the chicken, mix well and fry for 1 minute. Stir 2 more teaspoons of fajita spice mix into the mixture and fry for a further 2 minutes until the chicken is piping hot and aromatic. Add 2 tablespoons of cold water and cook for 2–3 minutes until the water reduces and you have a thick sauce.

7. Serve the fajita filling sizzling hot alongside the tortillas, Cheddar, avocado, salsa and soured cream for everyone to roll their own fajitas or stuff them yourself with the filling and any of your favourite additions. If you like the tortillas warm, pop them into a warm oven 5 minutes before serving.

NUTRITIONAL INFORMATION
(per serving)

Calories	Carbs
334	16g
Total Fat	**Protein**
21g	25g

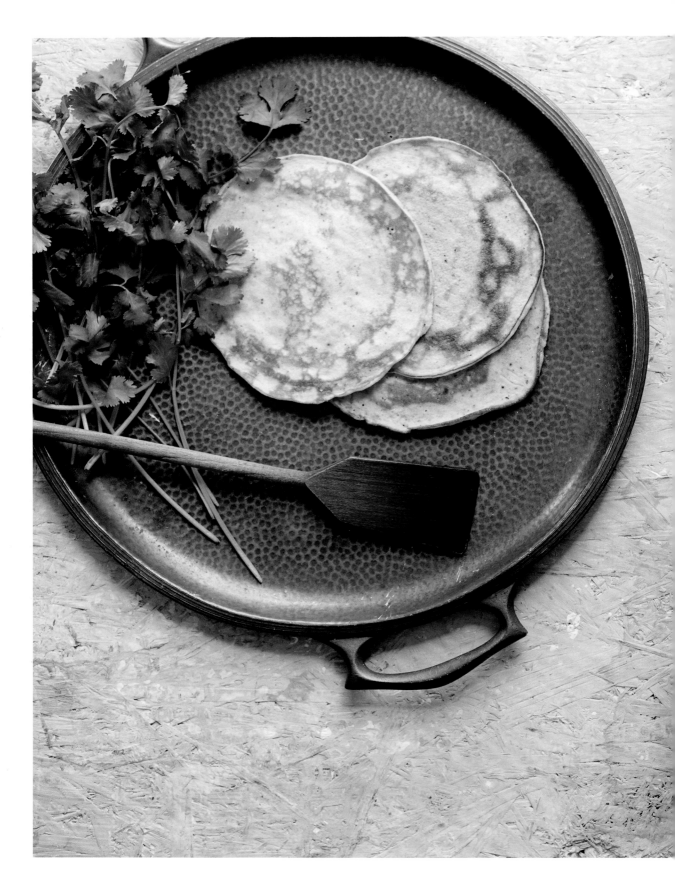

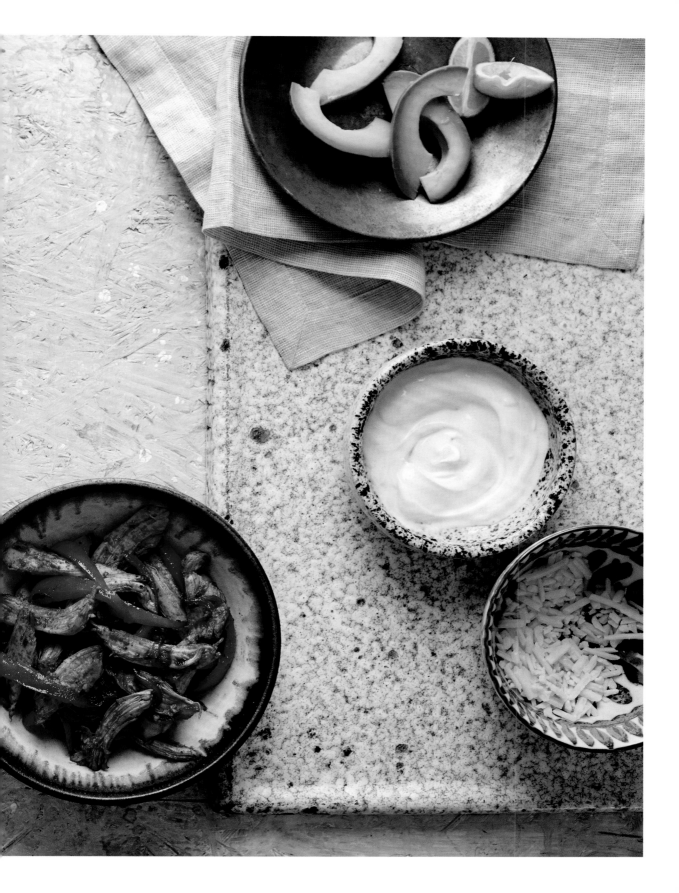

coconut chicken nuggets with a tomato and sweet paprika sauce

This is healthy fast-food at its finest, with no nasty additives or mytery ingredients. Simple to make, with a delicious crisp coating, it's hard to believe how low in carbs these chicken nuggets are. Great for the whole family, serve them straight from the oven with a side salad, some sweet potato wedges and the tomato and sweet paprika sauce.

If you don't have a food processor, buy the chicken already minced – you can ask a butcher to do this for you.

The tomato and sweet paprika sauce works wonderfully with the chicken nuggets. You can make it a day or two ahead and keep it in the fridge, or make it while the nuggets are baking and serve it warm. The longer you let it stand or chill, the more flavoursome it will be.

 4   **15 MINS**   **15–20 MINS**

For the chicken nuggets

2 large skinless and boneless chicken breasts (about 400g) or 400g minced chicken

2 garlic cloves, finely chopped

60g almond flour

½ tsp smoked paprika

½ tsp salt

¼ tsp cracked black pepper

1 large egg yolk, beaten

45g unsweetened desiccated coconut

120g coconut oil, plus extra for greasing

continues...

1. Preheat the oven to 200°C/400°F/gas mark 6.

2. Put the chicken breasts and garlic in a food processor and blitz on high speed for 10–15 seconds until the mixture has a paste-like texture. (If you are using minced chicken, mix it with the garlic in a bowl.)

3. In a separate bowl, combine 1 tablespoon of the almond flour with the paprika, salt, pepper and egg yolk. Tip in the chicken and garlic and mix until fully combined.

4. On a separate surface or baking sheet, roughly mix together the desiccated coconut and remaining almond flour.

5. Take 2 teaspoons of the chicken mix and roll it into a ball, then roll it in the coconut and almond mix to coat. Repeat with the rest of the chicken mixture.

6. Melt the coconut oil in a pan over high heat and cook the balls in batches on each side for 3–4 minutes until golden brown.

continues...

For the tomato and
sweet paprika sauce

2 tbsp olive oil

**½ medium red onion
(110g), very finely
chopped**

**2 garlic cloves, finely
chopped**

**1 x 400g tin chopped
tomatoes**

3 tsp sweet paprika

sea salt

7. Transfer the fried balls to a greased baking sheet and bake in the oven for 4–5 minutes until cooked through (cut one in half to check – the flesh should be white with no pink raw bits. If it isn't quite cooked, pop them all back into the oven for a further 4 minutes, then check again). Once cooked through, remove from oven and allow to sit for 5 minutes before serving.

8. Once the balls are in the oven, start making the tomato and sweet paprika sauce. Heat the olive oil in a pan over medium heat. Add the onion and garlic and cook for 4–5 minutes, stirring frequently, until softened.

9. Stir in the tomatoes and sweet paprika, then reduce to low heat and simmer for 8 minutes until the sauce has thickened. Season with salt to taste.

10. Serve the chicken balls with a large side salad and the sauce. You can keep any leftover sauce in a sealed container in the fridge for up to 5 days.

NUTRITIONAL INFORMATION
(per serving)

nuggets		*tomato sauce*	
Calories	**Carbs**	**Calories**	**Carbs**
635	7g	27	8g
Total Fat	**Protein**	**Total Fat**	**Protein**
55g	35g	1g	2g

stuffed turkey breast with garlic, nuts and olives

A simple, lean and succulent dish that's packed with flavour, and a very blood sugar-friendly and healthy way to add some pizzazz to the humble turkey.

This would be delicious served up with side dishes such as my pan-fried Brussels sprouts (see page 91) and some wok-fried greens in butter, or my Roasted Mediterranean vegetable couscous (see page 90).

 4   **15 MINS**   **35 MINS, PLUS COOLING**

500g skinless and boneless
 turkey breast

70g pitted green olives

50g walnuts

50g Brazil nuts

5 basil leaves

10 coriander leaves

4 garlic cloves, peeled

a pinch of cracked black
 pepper

½ tsp sea salt

1 tsp olive oil

1. Preheat the oven to 200°C/400°F/gas mark 6.

2. Place the turkey breast on a chopping board and carefully butterfly it by simply cut it down the middle but not quite all the way through, then open out the two pieces rather like opening a book.

3. Put the olives, walnuts, Brazil nuts, basil, coriander, garlic, pepper and salt in a blender or food processor and blitz until finely chopped with a paste-like consistency.

4. Spread the paste evenly over the inside of the turkey, then roll up the turkey breast lengthways until it is closed over the paste and tightly wrapped.

5. Drizzle a sheet of foil with the olive oil and place the turkey on top. Wrap the foil tightly around the turkey roll, twisting the ends to seal the package, and put it in a baking tin, then roast in the oven for 35 minutes.

6. Remove from the oven and allow to rest for 20 minutes before opening the foil.

7. If you like, you can sear the turkey on a griddle pan to give it a chargrilled effect.

8. Serve with your favourite seasonal side dishes.

NOTE: In this recipe, I use 500g turkey breast, but if you buy a bigger breast, adjust the cooking time accordingly. If you like, you can garnish the turkey roll with some chopped coriander leaves and toasted nuts.

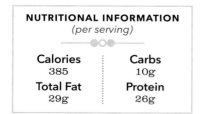

NUTRITIONAL INFORMATION
(per serving)

Calories	Carbs
385	10g
Total Fat	**Protein**
29g	26g

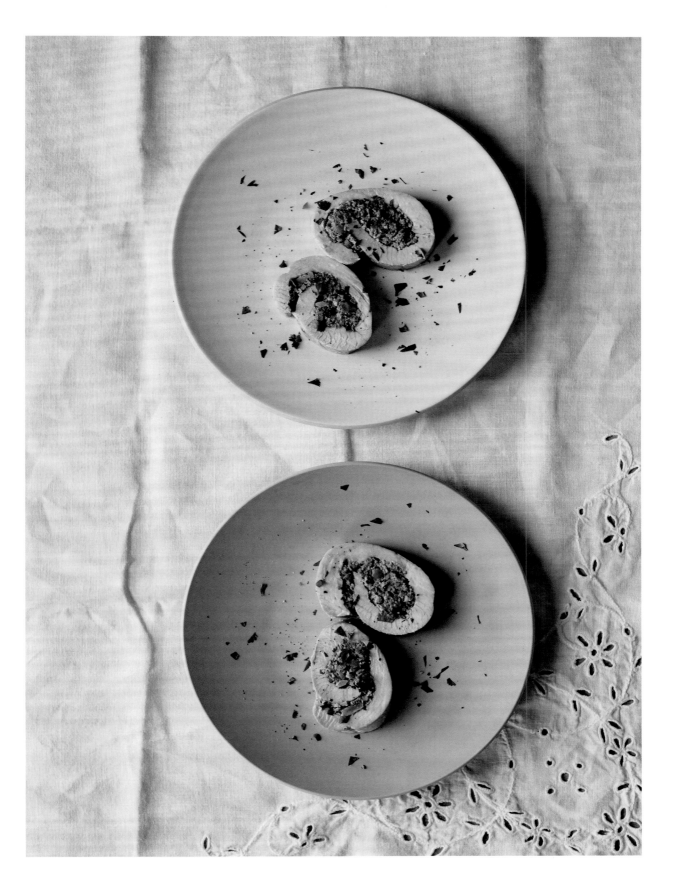

slow-roasted salt and pepper pulled pork

This is a real showstopper, perfect for a gathering of friends or family. Cooking the meat for five hours at a low heat creates the most divine and buttery pulled pork. It is melt-in-your-mouth, shout-from-the-rooftops delicious and it's well worth heading to your local butcher for a good piece of meat – in fact, get the best-quality meat you can afford.

The pork is also amazing as leftovers mixed with some fried onions, green pepper, ginger and sweet chilli for an Asian twist.

 4   5–10 MINS   APPROX. 5 HOURS 10 MINS, PLUS RESTING

1 tbsp olive oil

about 1.15kg pork loin shoulder or belly

sea salt and cracked black pepper

1. Preheat the oven to 220°C/425°F/gas mark 7 and grease a baking tray with a little of the olive oil.

2. Coat the meat generously with more olive oil, rubbing it all over the fat and skin, then sprinkle it with a generous layer of salt and pepper.

3. Put the meat in a roasting tin and cook in the oven for 10 minutes, then reduce the heat to 140°C/275°F/gas mark 1 and cook for 4½–5 hours, basting the meat with the juices from the tin every hour or so and turning the meat a few times.

4. Remove the crackling from the pork carefully and set aside to cool (allow the meat to rest for at least 15 minutes). Using two forks, pull the meat apart.

5. Serve the pork straightaway with large pieces of crackling, or cover with foil and put in the fridge once cool, until needed. Eat within 2 days.

NOTES: You can make this recipe with pork loin or belly. Both are delicious, but I think loin works the best.

If you want to serve this as a roast with vegetables, place whole garlic bulbs and your choice of roasted veg in with the pork around 40 minutes before the end of the meat's cooking time, and cook until roasted.

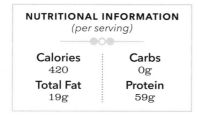

NUTRITIONAL INFORMATION
(per serving)

Calories	Carbs
420	0g
Total Fat	**Protein**
19g	59g

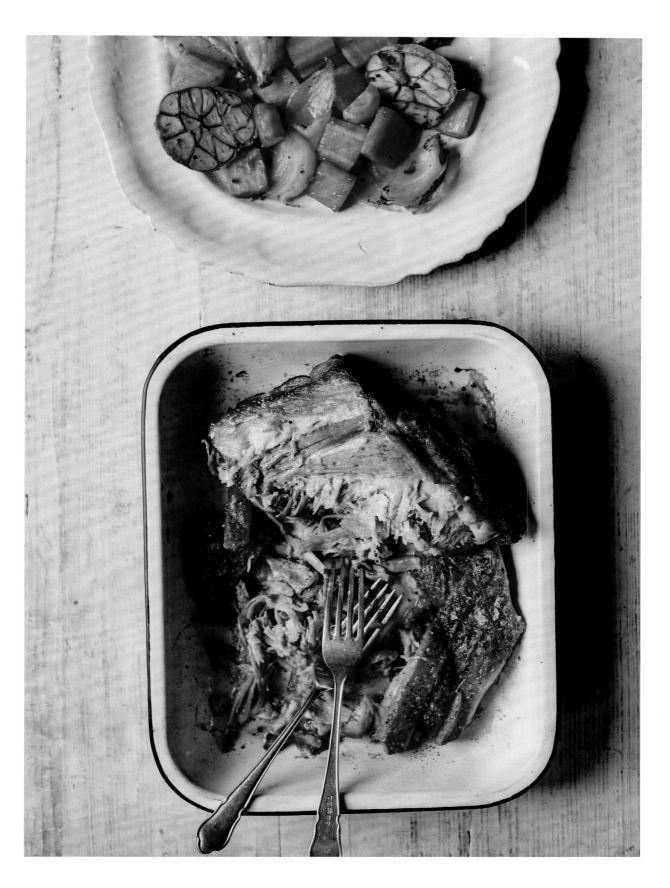

nutty mushroom risotto with bacon

This fresh, creamy, crunchy and meaty dish gives the same indulgent comfort as a normal rice-based risotto, but without the blood sugar high afterwards. I like to use chestnut mushrooms as they have a nuttier taste, but you can use any mushrooms. This is an incredibly tasty dish that goes from pan to plate in under 30 minutes. With its simple and nutritious ingredients, it is perfect for a casual weekday dinner with family or friends.

 4    **10 MINS**   **12–15 MINS**

1 large cauliflower (about 750g), cut into florets and tough stalks removed

2 garlic cloves, peeled

100g whole almonds

2 tsp coconut oil or olive oil

350g mushrooms, roughly chopped

3 spring onions (about 45g), finely chopped

3 rashers of unsmoked back bacon, sliced

1 x 200ml tin coconut milk

sea salt and cracked black pepper

coriander leaves, to garnish

grated Parmesan, to serve (optional)

1. Blitz the cauliflower and garlic in a food processor until very finely chopped, with the consistency of rice, then set aside. Alternatively, finely chop the garlic and coarsely grate the cauliflower on a box grater by hand.

2. Clean out the bowl of the food processor, add the almonds and pulse until roughly chopped.

3. Heat the oil in a pan over medium heat, add the mushrooms, spring onions and bacon and fry for 2 minutes, then stir in the almonds and cook for a further 2–3 minutes. Add the cauliflower and garlic rice and cook for 2–3 minutes.

4. Slowly pour in the coconut milk, stirring it in to combine, then reduce the heat and simmer for 6–7 minutes until thick and creamy. Season to taste with salt and pepper.

5. Serve garnished with coriander leaves and some grated Parmesan, if you like.

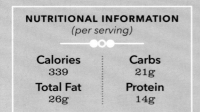

NUTRITIONAL INFORMATION
(per serving)

Calories	Carbs
339	21g
Total Fat	**Protein**
26g	14g

brilliant beef burgers

A simple burger recipe that contains none of the nasty additives found in most ready-made and fast-food burgers. These patties hold together beautifully and have a delicious texture and succulent meaty taste, and are best served straight from the oven with lettuce, tomato, gherkins, thinly sliced red onion and crumbled feta. This recipe is protein-packed and, of course, blood sugar-friendly. For accompaniments, opt for a small baked sweet potato or some of my Super seed bread (see page 198). They are also great cooked on the barbecue.

 4 10 MINS 15–20 MINS, PLUS COOLING

500g lean minced beef

1 medium onion (225g), finely diced

1 large egg, beaten

2 garlic cloves, crushed

2 beef stock cubes, crumbled

generous twist of cracked black pepper

2 tbsp ground coriander

1 tbsp smoked paprika

1 tbsp ground cumin

3 tbsp ground almonds

2 tbsp olive oil, plus extra for greasing

1. Preheat the oven to 220°C/425°F/gas mark 7, grease a baking tray and have a plate ready.

2. Put the minced beef, onion, egg, garlic, crumbled stock cubes, pepper, coriander, paprika, cumin and ground almonds in a large bowl. Massage the mince with clean hands, combining everything together evenly and to infuse all the flavours.

3. Take handfuls of the mince and mould them into 4 large (or 8 small) burger shapes. Carefully put the patties on the plate, then put them in the fridge, covered with cling film, for 30 minutes.

4. Heat a non-stick frying pan over medium heat, add the oil, then fry two burgers at a time for 3–4 minutes on each side until browned, to seal in the flavours. Carefully transfer to the baking tray and fry the other burgers until they have all been browned and sealed.

5. Cook the burgers in the oven for 6–7 minutes – if you'd like them to be on the rare side of medium, cook them for about 5 minutes. If you'd like them well cooked, cook for 8–10 minutes.

6. Serve straightaway with your preferred toppings and accompaniments.

NUTRITIONAL INFORMATION
(per serving)

Calories	Carbs
587	12g
Total Fat	**Protein**
44g	39g

Mrs P's cottage pie

Comforting, filling and full of flavour, this is a dish that I make often for family gatherings and dinner parties. It is comfort food personified, but without all the carbs. The topping's cheesy and baked to perfection with a creamy butternut and cauliflower mash that you can either make chunky or blend to a purée. If you'd prefer to completely cut out the carbs, use broccoli or aubergine instead of butternut, following the same method.

  6   **20 MINS**   **1 HOUR 30 MINS**

For the filling

2 tbsp olive oil

670g minced beef

190g onions, finely diced

65g mushrooms, finely diced

170g red pepper, deseeded and finely diced

2 garlic cloves, thinly sliced

1¼ tsp smoked paprika

1 beef stock cube, crumbled

1 tsp ground coriander

½ tsp ground cumin

2 x 400g tins chopped tomatoes

sea salt and black pepper

For the mash

500g butternut squash, peeled, deseeded and cubed

1 cauliflower (about 280g), cut into florets and tough stalks removed

100ml full-fat milk

50g butter

85g Cheddar cheese, grated

NUTRITIONAL INFORMATION
(per serving)

Calories	Carbs
447	22g
Total Fat	**Protein**
29g	31g

---

1. First, prepare the filling. Heat 1 tablespoon of the olive oil in a large saucepan over medium heat, add the mince and fry until browned. Remove with a slotted spoon and transfer to a plate.

2. In the same pan, heat the rest of the olive oil, add the onions, mushrooms and red pepper and fry for about 15 minutes, until soft. Add the garlic and cook for another 1–2 minutes, then return the cooked mince to the pan along with the smoked paprika, crumbled stock cube, ground coriander and cumin. Stir and cook for 3–4 minutes then add the chopped tomatoes.

3. Reduce the heat and simmer, uncovered, for about 30 minutes until thick. If the sauce still seems thin, increase the heat for a few minutes and cook until it has reduced and thickened. Season with salt and pepper to taste.

4. While the mince is simmering, prepare the mash. Cook the butternut squash and cauliflower in a pan of boiling water for 15–20 minutes until soft and tender. Drain, then mash with the milk, butter and 50g of the grated Cheddar.

5. Preheat the oven to 200°C/400°F/gas mark 6.

6. Spread the mince out evenly in a baking dish. Carefully place spoonfuls of the mash mixture on top, then spread it out with a fork. Bake in the oven for about 25 minutes then scatter with the remaining Cheddar, return to the oven and bake for a further 10 minutes until golden.

7. Serve immediately or allow to cool completely before covering with foil or cling film and storing it in the fridge until desired – it should be eaten within 2 days.

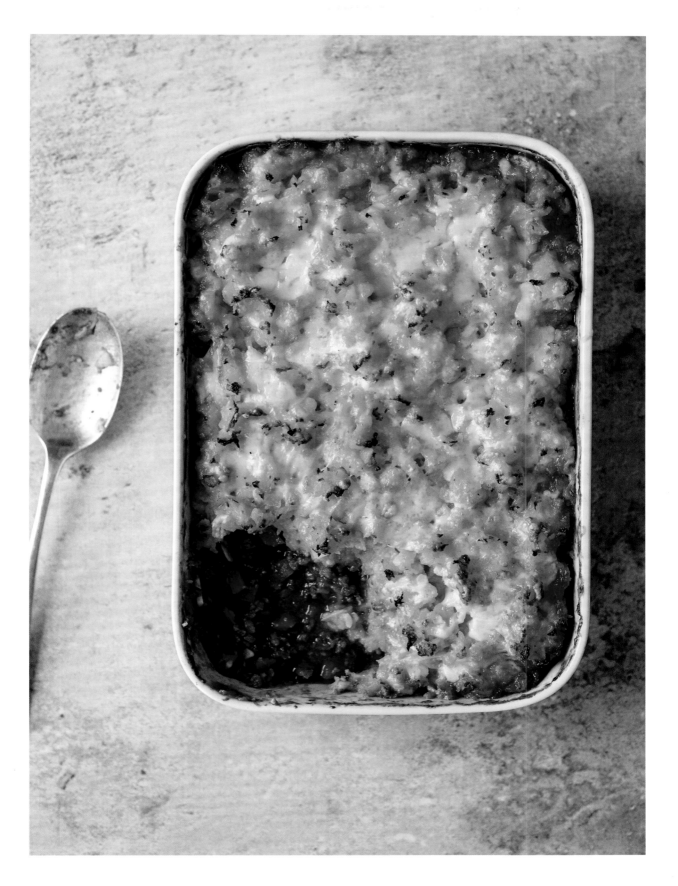

fiery steak stir-fry with spinach, pine nuts, onion and garlic

This is one dish that looks like it could have been served up by a world-class chef but in fact takes next to no time to cook and serve. It is filling, full of nutrients and protein and has all the delicious elements needed for a taste-tantalising supper.

The steak needs marinating for an hour prior to cooking, and the longer you can leave it marinating, the better the meat will taste.

 4   **10 MINS, PLUS 1 HOUR MARINATING**   **15 MINS**

1 tbsp smoked paprika

1 tsp red chilli flakes, plus extra to serve

450g rump steak, cut into 5mm wide strips

3 tbsp olive oil

85g pine nuts

1 large white onion (340g), thinly sliced

2 large garlic cloves, thinly sliced

100g small broccoli florets

200g spinach leaves

sea salt and cracked black pepper

1. Mix together the smoked paprika, chilli flakes and 1 teaspoon each of salt and pepper in a small bowl.

2. Coat the steak strips in 2 tablespoons of the olive oil in a large bowl, then tip in the spice mix.

3. Massage the meat with the spice mix and leave to marinate for at least 1 hour at room temperature, covered.

4. When you are ready to serve, dry-toast the pine nuts in a pan for about 3 minutes or until they start to colour. Tip out and set aside.

5. In the same pan heat the remaining olive oil, add the onion, garlic and broccoli and stir-fry for about 5 minutes.

6. Once the vegetables have softened and started to brown, add the spinach and cook for 1–2 minutes until wilted. Set the mixture aside in a warm bowl.

7. Place the same pan over high heat and fry the marinated meat for 1 minute on each side until browned all over. Add the stir-fried vegetables and pine nuts and fry for a further minute, making sure the ingredients are fully mixed. Add a sprinkle of chilli flakes, season with more salt and pepper if you like, and serve sizzling hot.

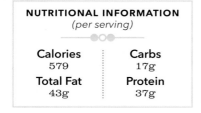

NUTRITIONAL INFORMATION
(per serving)

Calories	Carbs
579	17g
Total Fat	**Protein**
43g	37g

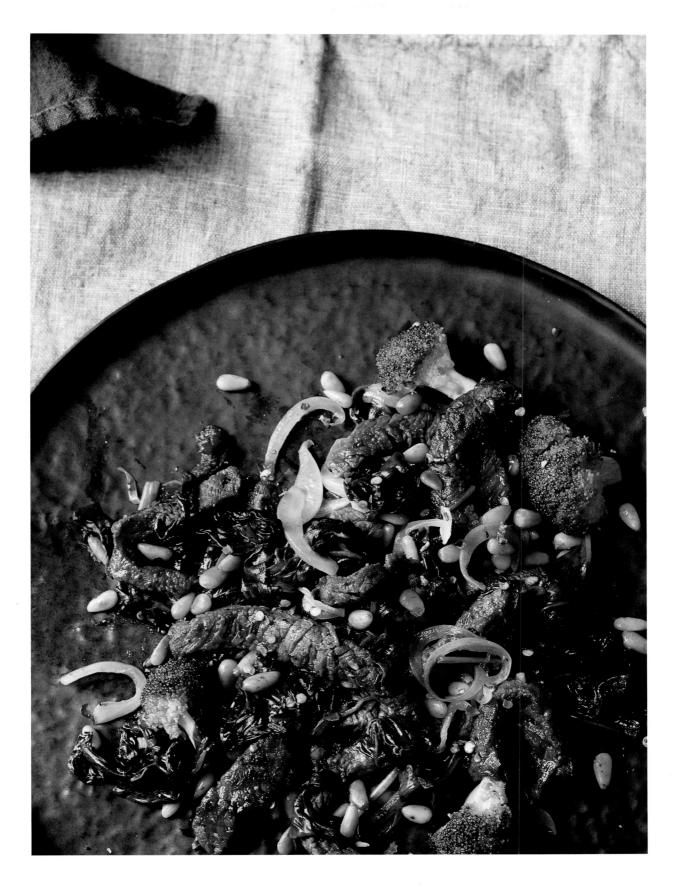

baked cod with a pistachio pesto crust

This dish is so quick and easy to make, packed with flavour and lots of nourishing goodness, with the added bonus of using easy-to-find ingredients that you can pick up from any local supermarket. There's hardly a carb in sight and it will make little impact to your blood sugar but leave you feeling immensely satisfied. The pistachio nuts work very well in the homemade pesto – I prefer them to pine nuts, but if you'd rather use pine nuts, please do so. It's delicious served with a salad, sweet potato chips or sautéed mushrooms.

 4   **10** MINS   **15** MINS

25g basil leaves

70ml cold-pressed extra-virgin olive oil, plus extra for greasing

1 tsp sea salt

4 garlic cloves, peeled

120g shelled unsalted pistachio nuts

4 cod fillets (about 700g total)

1. Preheat the oven to 200°C/400°F/gas mark 6 and grease a deep baking dish.

2. Put the basil leaves, olive oil, salt, garlic and pistachio nuts in a blender and blitz until broken down with a paste-like texture. You will probably have to use a spatula to scrape down the sides.

3. Put the cod fillets in the greased dish and spread about 2 tablespoons of pesto on top of each fish piece (if you have any pesto left over, put it in the fridge in a sealed container for another meal).

4. Place in the oven and cook for around 15 minutes until the top has browned and the cod is cooked through – the flesh should flake easily and be white all the way through, with no transparent flesh. Serve straightaway.

NUTRITIONAL INFORMATION
(per serving)

Calories	Carbs
444	10g
Total Fat	**Protein**
30g	36g

baked tarragon cod with lemon and garlic

This is the perfect dish if you are in a hurry. It is simple to make and full of nutritional goodness. Cod is such a wonderful fish as it is incredibly meaty and rich in omega-3 fatty acids, vitamins, protein and healthy fats, and you really couldn't find a dish lower in carbs.

This zesty dish is perfect for a weekday evening meal, or you could double or triple the recipe for a dinner with friends or family. Serve with a mixture of green seasonal vegetables smothered in butter and sprinkled with sea salt.

  2   **10 MINS**   **20 MINS**

2 tbsp olive oil

2 garlic cloves, finely diced

½ tsp sea salt

1 tbsp fresh lemon juice, plus 1 lemon, cut into about 6 wedges

4 tarragon stalks, leaves stripped and chopped, or use 1 tbsp dried tarragon

2 cod fillets

1. Preheat the oven to 200°C/400°F/gas mark 6.

2. Put the olive oil, garlic, salt, lemon juice and tarragon in a large bowl and whisk together well.

3. Dip the cod fillets into the mixture one at a time, to evenly coat all over.

4. Place the coated fillets in a deep baking dish and pour the remaining dipping mixture on top, then scatter the lemon wedges around the dish.

5. Cover with foil and cook in the oven for around 15 minutes then remove the foil and bake for a further 5 minutes until the fish flakes easily with a fork and the lemons have softened.

6. Remove from the oven and serve straightaway with the cooking juices drizzled over the fish and the softened lemon wedges.

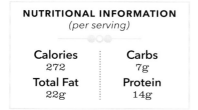

NUTRITIONAL INFORMATION
(per serving)

Calories	Carbs
272	7g
Total Fat	**Protein**
22g	14g

fish pie with a Parmesan, parsley and broccoli crust

This is ultimate comfort food and certainly one of my top five recipes in this book! It ticks every box for me: it's full of flavour, jam-packed with protein, good fats and lots of nutrients, and the great thing about this is that you can prepare it in advance, chill it for up to three days, or freeze it until needed. I like to make it as one large dish, but if you'd rather, you can serve it in individual pots, too.

This is perfect for any gathering of friends and family. Try serving it with green beans, steamed broccoli and garlic or some kale.

6   **15 MINS**   **1 HOUR**

For the parsley and broccoli crust

250g butternut squash, peeled and cut into rough chunks

400g broccoli, cut into florets and tough stalks removed

3 tsp butter

a handful of flat-leaf parsley, chopped

3 tbsp grated Parmesan

sea salt and cracked black pepper

continues...

1. Preheat the oven to 220°C/425°F/gas mark 7.

2. Start by making the parsley and broccoli crust. Put the butternut squash in a pan and cover with water. Bring to the boil and simmer for 10 minutes then add the broccoli and cook for a further 10–15 minutes until tender. Drain well, then mash in the dry pan with the butter, some seasoning and three-quarters of the chopped parsley. Set aside.

3. Now, start on the filling. Put the butter, spring onions, leeks and celery in a deep-sided pan over low heat and sweat, covered, for 3–4 minutes until softened.

4. Stir in the coconut flour using a wooden spoon, then gradually add the coconut milk and whisk until fully incorporated and there are no lumps in the mixture. Turn up the heat and cook until the mixture has reached boiling point, then reduce the heat and cook at a gentle simmer for 3–4 minutes, until the sauce has thickened.

5. Remove the pan from the heat and stir in the grated Cheddar, fish mix and peas, and season with salt and pepper.

continues...

NUTRITIONAL INFORMATION
(per serving)

Calories	Carbs
384	20g
Total Fat	**Protein**
26g	22g

For the filling

25g butter

2 spring onions (about 30g), roughly chopped

100g leeks, sliced

20g celery sticks, diced

25g coconut flour

1 x 400ml tin of coconut milk

50g Cheddar cheese, grated

420g boneless fish fillets, skinned and cut into 2.5cm chunks (I use a mix of cod, smoked haddock and salmon) and prawns

100g frozen or fresh peas

6. Pour the fish mixture into a baking dish and spoon the broccoli mash mixture on top, using a fork to level it out.

7. Pop into the oven and cook for 20 minutes. Preheat the grill.

8. After 20 minutes, carefully remove the pie from the oven, sprinkle over the Parmesan and the remaining parsley then place it under the hot grill to crisp up for 10 minutes.

9. Once bubbling and golden, remove from the grill and allow the dish to rest for 5 minutes before serving. Alternatively, allow it to fully cool before chilling it in the fridge. Fully covered, the pie will keep in the fridge for 2–3 days. You can also freeze it until needed.

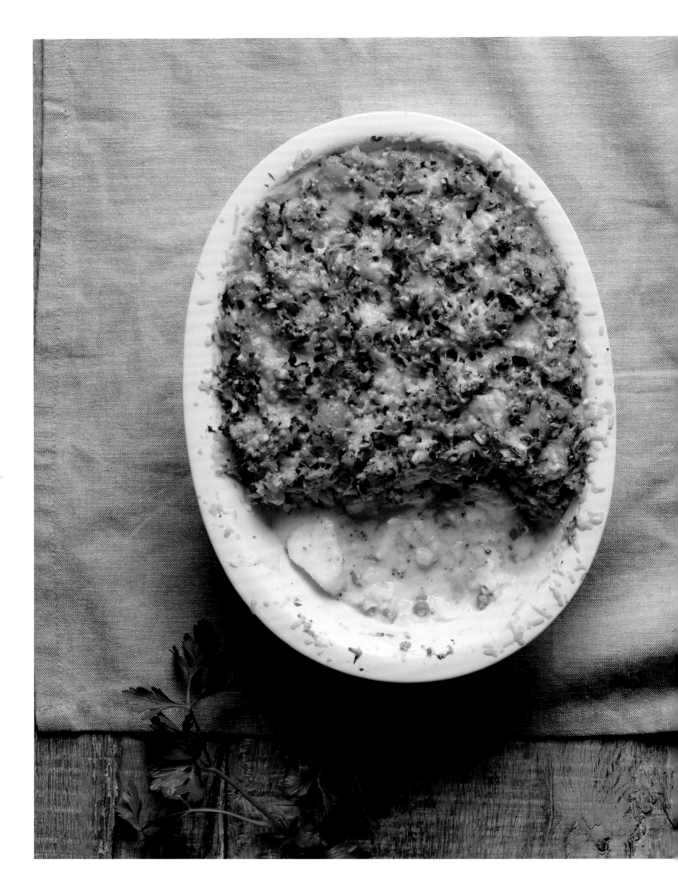

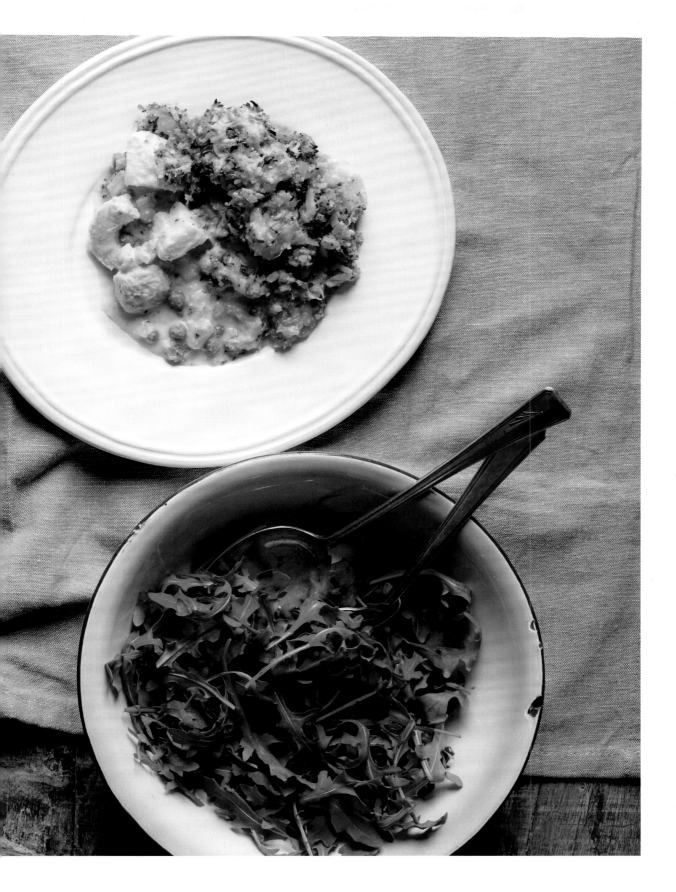

courgette 'spaghetti' with feta and a lemon yoghurt dressing

I understand the universal love for pasta, but for anyone with diabetes, it's such a high-carb conundrum.

Courgette 'spaghetti' isn't your glutenous pasta. It's fresher, filling and much better for you. This is a great, no-cook summer lunch or supper dish and would work wonderfully with added protein such as chicken, salmon or egg. Delicious and creamy, it's quick to make and will leave your taste buds tantalised!

 4 15 MINS

For the courgette 'spaghetti'

500g courgettes
1 tbsp olive oil
2 tbsp tahini paste
100g feta, crumbled
½ tsp rock salt or sea salt

For the lemon yoghurt dressing

juice of ½ lemon
100g full-fat plain yoghurt
cracked black pepper
coriander leaves, to garnish

1. Use a spiralizer (see Note on page 94) to create courgette noodles, or use a vegetable or julienne peeler, or a sharp knife to carefully cut the courgette into long thin strands.

2. Place the courgette spaghetti in a large bowl, pour in the olive oil and toss it through the courgette. Add the tahini, crumbled feta and salt. Using clean hands, combine everything to coat the courgette.

3. To make the yoghurt dressing, put the lemon juice, yoghurt, 2–3 tablespoons of water and some cracked black pepper in a bowl and stir well until smooth and runny.

4. Serve the courgette spaghetti straightaway, drizzled with a generous amount of lemon yoghurt dressing and garnished with coriander.

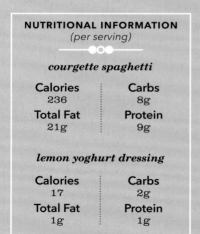

NUTRITIONAL INFORMATION
(per serving)

courgette spaghetti

Calories	Carbs
236	8g
Total Fat	**Protein**
21g	9g

lemon yoghurt dressing

Calories	Carbs
17	2g
Total Fat	**Protein**
1g	1g

roasted aubergine with kale pesto

Packed with nutrients, vitamins and lots of health-boosting goodness, this dish certainly excites the taste buds! Aubergine is a delicious and versatile vegetable that is incredibly nutritious and gives you a brilliant dose of dietary fibre. The kale pesto is the perfect accompaniment to the roasted aubergine, and the quantity below makes enough for there to be leftovers for another meal (keep it in a sealed container in the fridge for up to three days).

 2   **10** MINS   **25** MINS

1 large aubergine, halved lengthways

120ml olive oil, plus extra for drizzling

15 whole Brazil nuts

100g kale

15g basil leaves

60g pomegranate seeds

1 tbsp brined capers

sea salt and cracked black pepper

1. Preheat the oven to 190°C/375°F/gas mark 5.

2. Place the two aubergine halves on a baking sheet, score the cut surface in a criss-cross pattern with a sharp knife, drizzle with 1 tablespoon of olive oil and season with salt and pepper.

3. Roast the aubergine in the oven for about 25 minutes, until cooked through and tender.

4. Meanwhile, make the kale pesto. Blitz the Brazil nuts, 120ml olive oil, kale, ½ teaspoon of sea salt and the basil in a food processor until smooth and combined. You will probably have to use a spatula to scrape down the sides. Add more olive oil if it's not smooth enough and keep blending until it reaches your desired consistency. Have a taste and add more salt if needed.

5. Remove the aubergine from the oven, spoon about 1 tablespoon of the pesto over it and spread it to cover.

6. Sprinkle over the pomegranate seeds and capers and drizzle with some more olive oil if you wish. Serve straightaway.

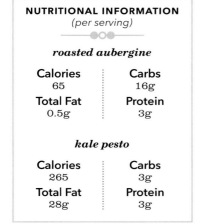

NUTRITIONAL INFORMATION
(per serving)

roasted aubergine

Calories	Carbs
65	16g
Total Fat	**Protein**
0.5g	3g

kale pesto

Calories	Carbs
265	3g
Total Fat	**Protein**
28g	3g

butternut squash and almond butter curry

This veggie curry has a thick and creamy sauce and lots of texture. It's also bursting with nutrients and vitamins. I love to add fresh coriander when I serve it, but if that doesn't take your fancy, just leave it out. You can use any nut butter you like, but I like the almond butter taste the most.

 4   **10 MINS**   **50 MINS**

2 tsp coconut oil

1 large white onion, finely chopped

500g butternut squash (about 340g), peeled, deseeded and cut into bite-sized cubes

½ tsp ground ginger

1½ tsp ground cumin

2 tsp garam masala

1 tsp ground turmeric

3 tbsp almond butter

1 tsp sea salt

1 x 400g tin chopped tomatoes

coriander leaves, to garnish

1. Melt the coconut oil in a deep pan over high heat. Add the onion and butternut squash and cook for 4–5 minutes until the onion has browned at the edges and turned translucent.

2. Add the ginger, cumin, garam masala and turmeric, coating the vegetables with the spices, and continue to cook for 2–3 minutes, stirring regularly with a wooden spoon, then add the almond butter and salt with 2 tablespoons of water and stir to combine, then add the chopped tomatoes and 400ml water.

3. Stir and bring to the boil then turn down the heat and simmer, uncovered, for about 40 minutes until the sauce has thickened and the butternut squash is soft.

4. Serve straightaway with cauliflower rice, if you like (see recipe on page 133 and nutritional note on page 132), garnished with coriander or allow to cool and keep in the fridge in a sealed container for up to 3 days, or pop into the freezer.

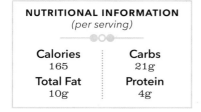

NUTRITIONAL INFORMATION
(per serving)

Calories	Carbs
165	21g
Total Fat	**Protein**
10g	4g

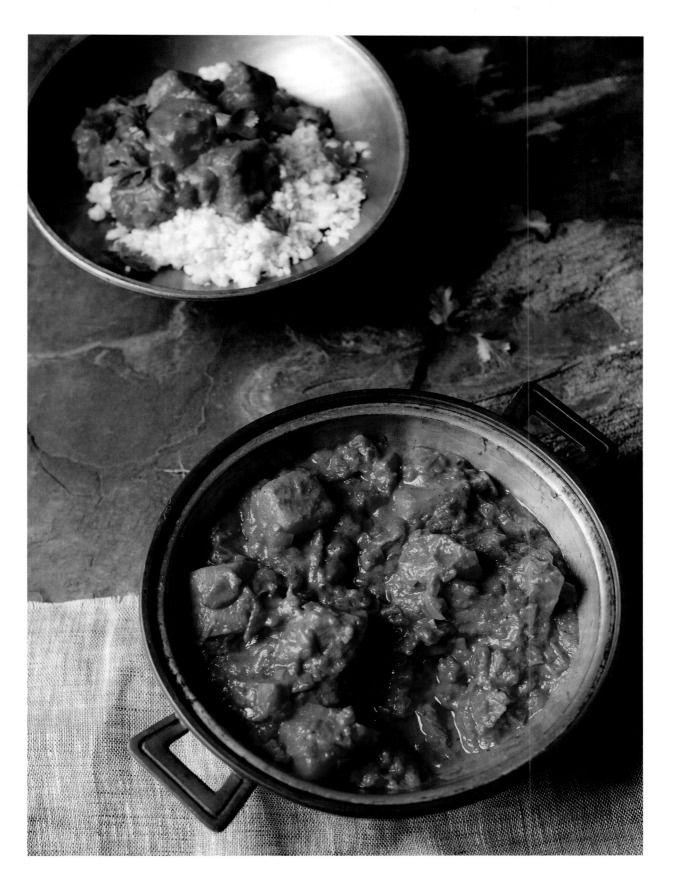

cheesy cauliflower pizza

If you like cheese this is one recipe that you'll want to bookmark. It's so easy to make and you can choose whatever topping you prefer. I suggest adding lots of greens, roasted veggies and grated Cheddar. You could also add shredded chicken, prawns or tuna for extra protein. I've included three of my own favourite toppings to get you started.

It's important to drain the cauliflower thoroughly; if you don't do this, the pizza won't stay together or will be very soggy.

 3   **15** MINS   **30** MINS, PLUS STANDING

450g cauliflower, cut into florets and tough stalks removed

120g mature Cheddar cheese, finely grated

100g mozzarella, grated

100g ground almonds

1 tsp each of ground sea salt and cracked black pepper

2 tsp mixed dried herbs

1 large egg, beaten

For a tomato, cheese and basil topping

1 x 400g tin chopped tomatoes

50g mature Cheddar cheese, grated

a few basil leaves

continues...

1. Preheat the oven to 220°C/425°F/gas mark 7.

2. Blitz the cauliflower florets in a food processor until they have a rice-like consistency. Alternatively, use a box grater to grate the cauliflower by hand.

3. Put the grated cauliflower in a piece of muslin, or a sieve lined with kitchen paper set over a bowl and allow all the water to drain away.

4. Transfer the cauliflower to a large bowl, add all the other ingredients and mould into a ball.

5. Split the ball into three. Press each one onto a baking sheet into a circular pizza shape (I like to use a non-stick sheet, but if you do not have a non-stick one, grease the baking sheet or line it with some greaseproof paper).

6. Bake for 12–14 minutes until the pizza bases are cooked and turning golden brown.

continues...

For a ham, fig and
 rocket topping

**2 slices of butcher's
 unsmoked ham (50g),
 cut into strips**

**1 fig, stalk removed, cut
 into thin slices**

**a handful of rocket (add
 this after cooking and
 just before serving)**

For a chicken, red onion
 and courgette topping

**a handful of shredded
 cooked chicken**

**½ red onion, thinly sliced
 (about 50g)**

**½ courgette, thinly sliced
 (about 80g)**

7. Scatter your preferred topping evenly over the
pizza bases then pop the pizzas back into the oven for
15 minutes until fully cooked and golden.

8. Carefully remove from the oven and let the pizzas
stand for 15 minutes before serving with some fresh
salad.

NOTE: When buying chopped tomatoes in a tin,
always check the tin label to make sure there is no
added sugar or salt.

NUTRITIONAL INFORMATION
(per serving)

tomato, cheese, basil		*ham, fig, rocket*		*chicken, red onion, courgette*	
Calories 925	**Carbs** 22g	**Calories** 300	**Carbs** 19g	**Calories** 600	**Carbs** 18g
Total Fat 46g	**Protein** 35g	**Total Fat** 44g	**Protein** 35g	**Total Fat** 43g	**Protein** 39g

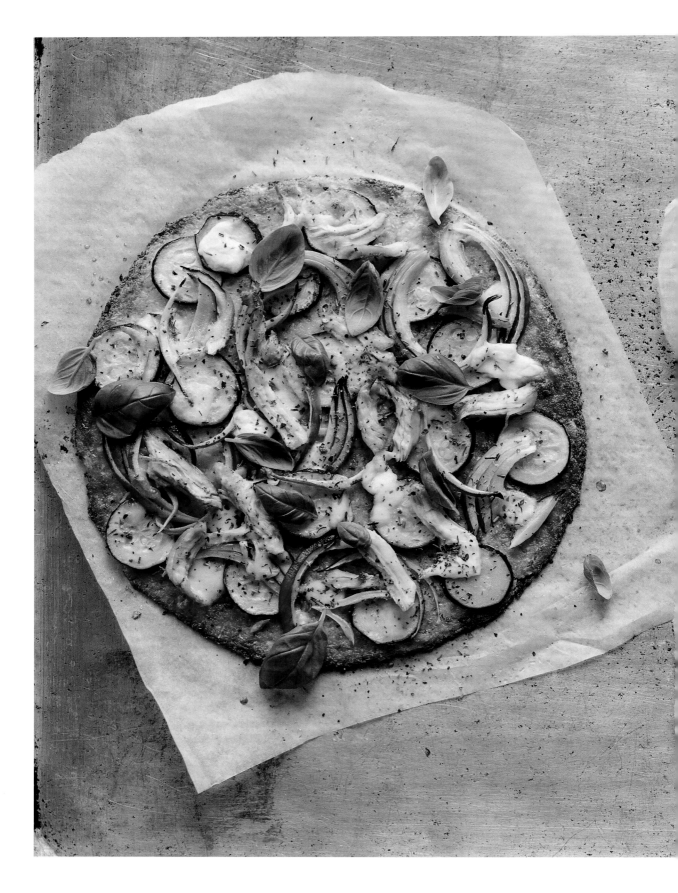

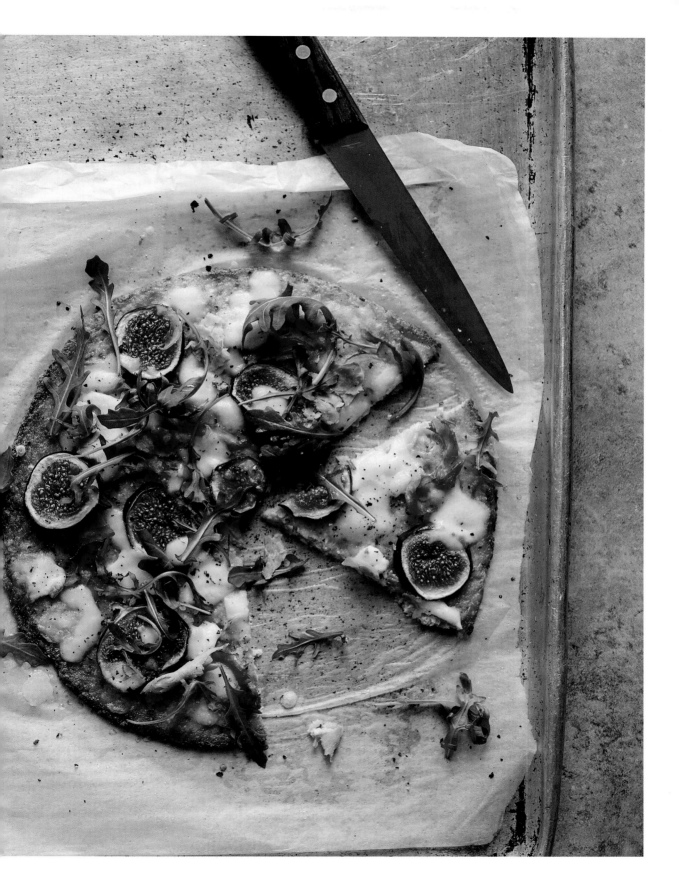

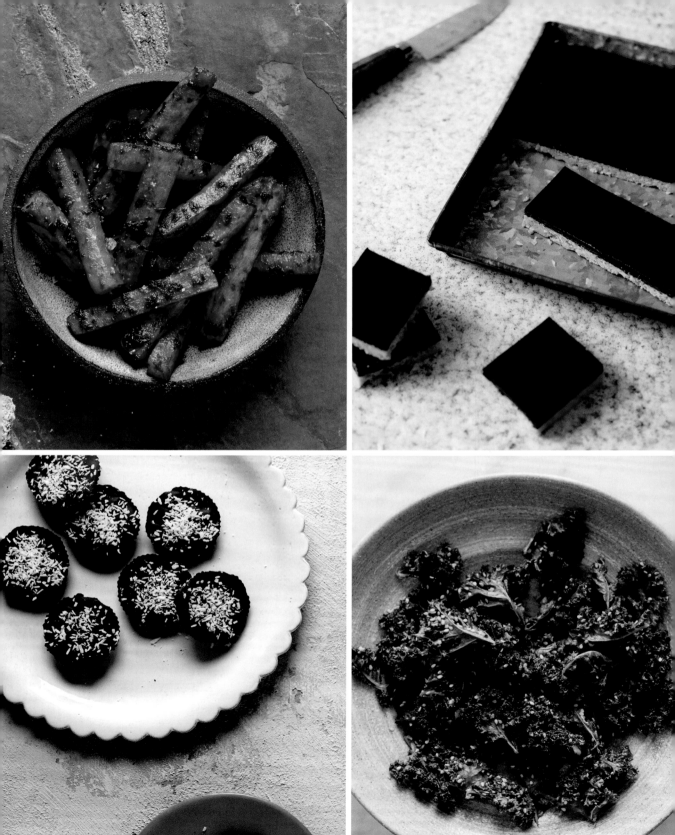

Side dishes & snacks

Roasted broccoli with sun-dried
tomatoes, capers and mozzarella
172

Crushed creamy peas with basil
174

Roasted cauliflower and Parmesan
bites with a soured cream
and chive dip
175

Crunchy garlic and chilli prawns
176

Pork, apple and sage savoury bites
178

FRIES FOUR WAYS
Garlic and rosemary
sweet potato fries
180

Smoky carrot fries
180

Cheesy courgette fries
181

Peppery avocado fries
181

Sesame kale crisps
184

Sea salt and lemon zest almonds
186

Cracked pepper and sea salt
multi-seed crackers
187

Chia and chocolate orange
energy balls
188

Peanut butter cups
190

Chocolate coconut cups
191

Chocolate shortbread squares
194

roasted broccoli with sun-dried tomatoes, capers and mozzarella

Broccoli is a wonderful vegetable that can be cooked in so many ways. In this really simple dish roasting it adds flavour and crunch and brings the broccoli to life. While this is great served on its own, it also works as a side dish, hot or cold, with baked lemon salmon or with roast chicken (see page 128). A brilliant dish to share, vibrant, flavour-packed and low in carbs. What more could you wish for?

 4   5 MINS   36 MINS

350g broccoli, cut into florets and tough stalks removed

2 tbsp olive oil

sea salt and cracked black pepper

50g sun-dried tomatoes from a jar, drained and roughly chopped

2 tbsp brined capers

60g mozzarella, chopped

1. Preheat the oven to 220°C/425°F/gas mark 7.

2. Spread the broccoli florets out on a roasting dish, drizzle with the olive oil and season with salt and pepper. Bake in the oven for 30 minutes.

3. Remove from the oven and evenly mix in the sun-dried tomatoes and scatter over the capers. Scatter the mozzarella on top.

4. Pop back in the oven for a further 6 minutes until the mozzarella has melted.

5. Carefully remove from the oven and serve straightaway or allow to cool, then cover and chill in the fridge to eat cold later.

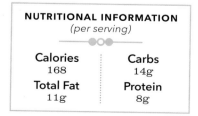

NUTRITIONAL INFORMATION
(per serving)

Calories	Carbs
168	14g
Total Fat	**Protein**
11g	8g

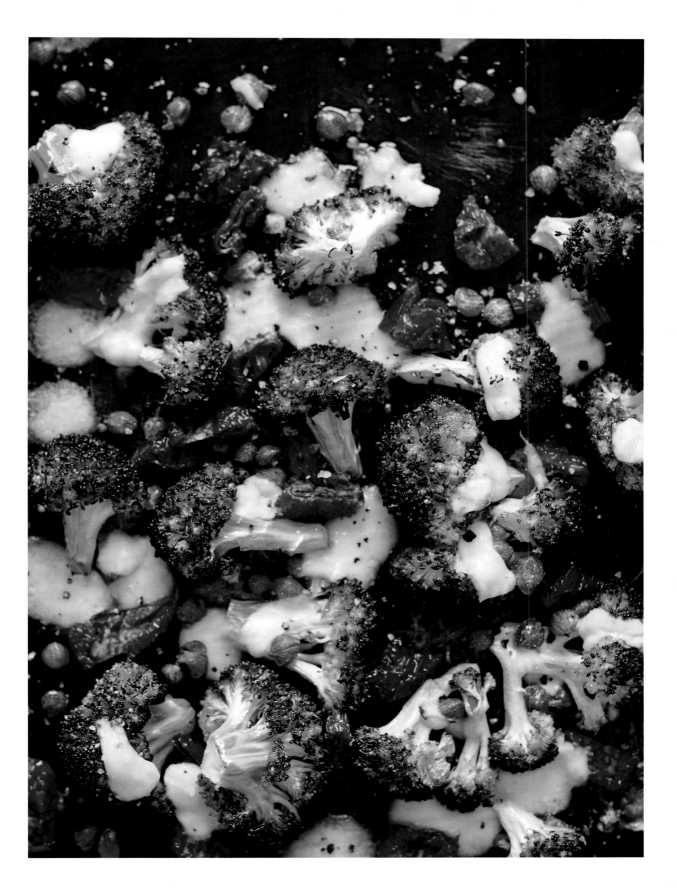

crushed creamy peas with basil

Great for the whole family, this dish is fresh, flavour-packed, low carb and, most importantly, blood sugar-friendly. This is my own take on the popular pea and mint combination; the peas are creamy and flavoursome with the subtle hint of basil and sea salt. My favourite way to serve these peas is with some baked fish, preferably cod, as the two go beautifully together.

If you don't eat dairy, you can replace the crème fraîche with plain or coconut yoghurt.

 4   **5 MINS**   **6 MINS**

200g frozen garden peas

8 basil leaves

½ tsp sea salt

2 tbsp crème fraîche (add 1 more tbsp if you like it extra creamy)

½ tsp sea salt

1. Bring a pan of water to boil over a high heat with the frozen peas in it. Cover and reduce the heat, then simmer for 3–4 minutes until cooked.

2. Drain and rinse under cold running water to cool (alternatively, put them in a bowl of iced water), and to help retain the vibrant green colour.

3. Put the peas, basil, salt and crème fraîche in a blender or food processor. Pulse 4–5 times until crushed and creamy but still textured.

4. Reheat in a pan over low heat if you want to serve them hot, or serve cold.

NOTE: If you don't have a blender, mash the peas by hand, chop the basil leaves finely and stir in the crème fraîche.

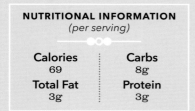

NUTRITIONAL INFORMATION
(per serving)

Calories	Carbs
69	8g
Total Fat	**Protein**
3g	3g

roasted cauliflower and Parmesan bites with a soured cream and chive dip

A twist on classic cauliflower cheese. These bites are a simple and delicious finger food, one to hand around at a party, take to a picnic or have in a beautiful serving bowl at a barbecue. They also make a great addition to a salad.

 4   15 MINS   37 MINS

For the cauliflower and Parmesan bites

315g cauliflower, cut into small florets and tough stalks removed

2 tbsp olive oil

2 large eggs

50g Cheddar cheese, grated

1½ tsp wholegrain mustard

2 tbsp freshly grated Parmesan

½ tsp cracked black pepper

For the soured cream and chive dip

4 tbsp soured cream

a handful of chives, finely chopped

a pinch each of sea salt and cracked black pepper

½ tsp grated lemon zest and 1 tbsp juice

1. Preheat the oven to 220°C/425°F/gas mark 7.

2. Place the cauliflower florets on a baking tray, drizzle with the olive oil and roast in the oven for 15 minutes.

3. Meanwhile, whisk the eggs in a bowl and add the grated Cheddar and the mustard.

4. Take out the cauliflower and pour the egg mixture over it in the baking tray. Make sure all the florets are coated. Return to the oven and, after 2 minutes, stir the mixture, scraping up any residual egg on the bottom of the tray and covering all the florets. Return the tray to the oven, reduce the temperature to 200°C/400°F/gas mark 6 and roast the cauliflower for a further 15 minutes until golden.

5. Carefully remove from oven, scatter with the grated Parmesan and cracked black pepper and cook for a further 5 minutes. Once cooked, leave to cool a little.

6. Meanwhile, combine the soured cream, chives, salt and pepper in a small serving bowl, mixing together well. Add the lemon zest and juice and serve straightaway with the cauliflower bites.

NUTRITIONAL INFORMATION
(per serving)

cauliflower bites		*soured cream dip*	
Calories	Carbs	Calories	Carbs
182	5g	32	1g
Total Fat	Protein	Total Fat	Protein
15g	9g	4g	0.5g

crunchy garlic and chilli prawns

These crunchy, crisp paprika prawns are very simple to make and are the perfect canapé, snack or addition to a salad. They go perfectly with my Tomato and sweet paprika sauce (see page 144) or Avocado and chilli cream dip (see page 125).

Buy freshly cooked and peeled prawns from a fishmonger if you can, or the chilled aisle of the supermarket. If you are using frozen prawns, be aware that they will contain added water that could make them soggy.

 4   **10 MINS**   **20 MINS**

2 large egg whites

75g ground almonds

1 tsp chilli powder

3 garlic cloves, crushed

½ tsp sea salt (optional)

¼ tsp cracked black pepper (optional)

160g raw peeled king prawns

1. Preheat the oven to 200°C/400°F/gas mark 6 and line a baking tray with foil or baking parchment.

2. Whisk the egg whites in a large, clean bowl, until fluffy and starting to stiffen.

3. Put the ground almonds, chilli powder, garlic and salt and pepper, if using, on a plate and mix together until fully combined and evenly spread out.

4. Using clean hands, dip the prawns, one at a time, into the egg-white mix, then place them straight into the dry mixture to coat them. Place on the baking sheet and repeat until you have coated all the prawns.

5. Cook in the oven for about 20 minutes until golden brown (keep an eye on them).

6. As soon as they are golden brown and crisp, serve them straightaway or allow to cool and eat cold.

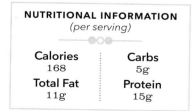

NUTRITIONAL INFORMATION
(per serving)

Calories	Carbs
168	5g
Total Fat	**Protein**
11g	15g

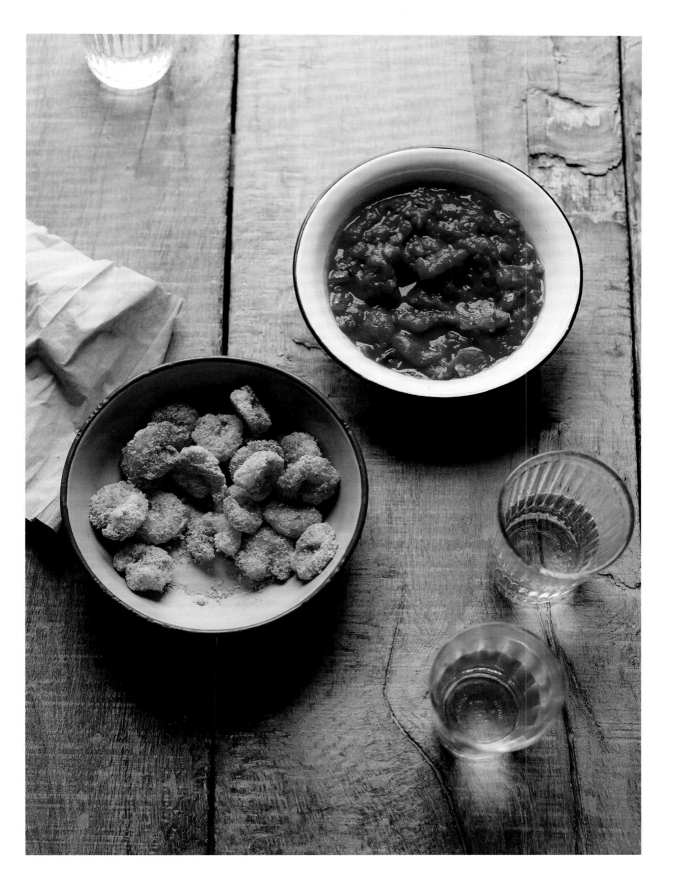

pork, apple and sage savoury bites

These mini pork, sage and apple savoury bites are the perfect taste-tantaliser. Served hot or cold, they are great as party finger food, or as a side dish to a weekend roast dinner.

 4   15 MINS   40 MINS

450g sausage meat (buy this from your butcher, or if you are buying from a supermarket be aware of added ingredients and go for 450g organic minced pork if possible)

1 small white onion (about 110g), finely chopped

2 tbsp ground almonds

1 apple (about 150g), cored and finely chopped

½ tsp each of sea salt and cracked black pepper

2 tsp dried sage

1 large egg, beaten

1. Preheat the oven to 200°C/400°F/gas mark 6.

2. Put all the ingredients in a large bowl and use your hands to mix them together until evenly combined.

3. Roll the mixture into 12–14 bite-sized balls, place them on a baking tray and bake in the oven for 25 minutes, then turn the balls and place them back in the oven for a further 15 minutes until golden brown and fully cooked through.

4. Serve hot or allow to cool and store in the fridge to eat cold. Eat within 3 days.

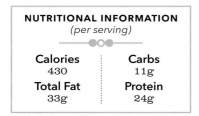

NUTRITIONAL INFORMATION
(per serving)

Calories	Carbs
430	11g
Total Fat	**Protein**
33g	24g

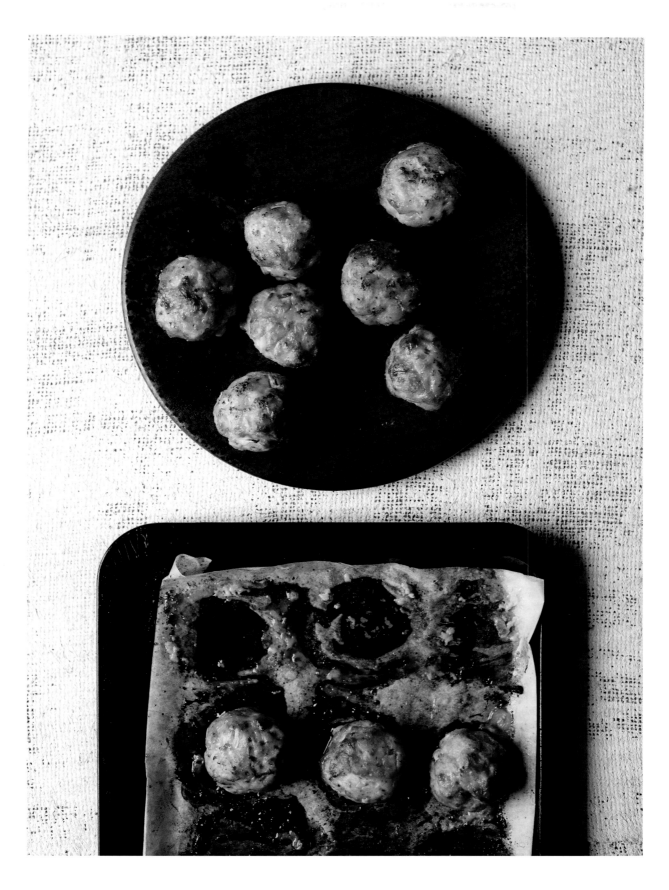

Fries four ways
garlic and rosemary sweet potato fries

These sweet potato fries are a great substitute for conventional potato chips, and are perfect for the whole family. Serve as a side dish to a homemade burger (see page 151) or as a savoury snack. Sweet potatoes are higher in carbohydrates than most vegetables so should be enjoyed in moderation.

 4   **10** MINS   🍲 **25** MINS

1 large sweet potato (about 280g), cut into fries

2 tsp olive oil

2 tsp chopped rosemary

1 garlic clove, crushed

sea salt and cracked black pepper

1. Preheat the oven to 220°C/425°F/gas mark 7 and line a baking sheet with greaseproof paper.

2. Place the fries in a large bowl with the oil, rosemary, crushed garlic and some salt and pepper. Mix well to coat.

3. Spread the fries evenly over the baking sheet and bake for about 25 minutes until crispy with a soft centre.

NUTRITIONAL INFORMATION	
(per serving)	
Calories	Carbs
123	15g
Total Fat	Protein
7g	2g

smoky carrot fries

These smoky carrot fries are a perfect, easy and yummy side dish or savoury snack: a totally guilt-free alternative to traditional potato fries.

 4   **10** MINS   🍲 **20–25** MINS

2 large carrots (about 145g)

2 tbsp olive oil

1 tbsp dried parsley

2 tsp smoked paprika

1 tsp sea salt

1. Preheat the oven to 220°C/425°F/gas mark 7 and line a baking sheet with greaseproof paper.

2. Top and tail the carrots, then cut them in half widthways and slice lengthways into about 32 fries.

3. Put the fries in a large bowl with the olive oil, parsley, smoked paprika and sea salt and stir to coat.

4. Spread the fries evenly over the baking sheet and bake for 20–25 minutes until golden and crispy.

NUTRITIONAL INFORMATION	
(per serving)	
Calories	Carbs
78	5g
Total Fat	Protein
7g	1g

cheesy courgette fries

A delicious, simple, low-carb alternative to potato fries. Great as a snack, a side dish or a healthier alternative to toasted fingers to dip into a boiled egg.

 4   10 MINS   20 MINS

1 large courgette (about 165g), topped and tailed

100g Parmesan, grated

2 tbsp ground almonds

1 tsp dried basil

1 tsp garlic powder

2 large eggs

sea salt and black pepper

NUTRITIONAL INFORMATION	
(per serving)	
Calories	Carbs
196	5g
Total Fat	Protein
14g	15g

1. Preheat the oven to 220°C/425°F/gas mark 7 and line a baking sheet with greaseproof paper.

2. Cut the courgette in half widthways and slice lengthways into fries. You should end up with around 32 fries.

3. Put the Parmesan, ground almonds, basil, garlic powder and some salt and pepper into a bowl with the courgette fries and mix well until combined. Beat the eggs in a separate bowl.

4. Coat the courgette fries, one at a time, in the beaten egg, then in the dry mix. Place each fry on the baking sheet. Repeat until all the fries are coated.

5. Bake for about 20 minutes until golden and crispy.

peppery avocado fries

Crispy and buttery yumminess: these addictive fries are actually good for you.

 4   10 MINS   15 MINS

2 avocados, stones removed

4 tbsp ground almonds

¼ tsp garlic powder

1 tsp sea salt

2 tsp cracked black pepper

1 large egg, beaten

NUTRITIONAL INFORMATION	
(per serving)	
Calories	Carbs
267	12g
Total Fat	Protein
24g	7g

1. Preheat the oven to 220°C/425°F/gas mark 7 and line a baking sheet with greaseproof paper.

2. Scoop out the flesh from each half avocado as one piece and place flat-side down on a chopping board. Cut the flesh widthways into fries, then each slice in half lengthways.

3. Put the ground almonds in a bowl, combine the garlic powder, salt and pepper in another bowl, and put the beaten egg in a third bowl.

4. Coat the avocado fries, one at a time, in the almonds, then the egg, then the garlic powder mix, pressing so that the crumbs stick. Place each fry on the baking sheet and repeat until all the fries are coated.

5. Bake for about 15 minutes or until golden.

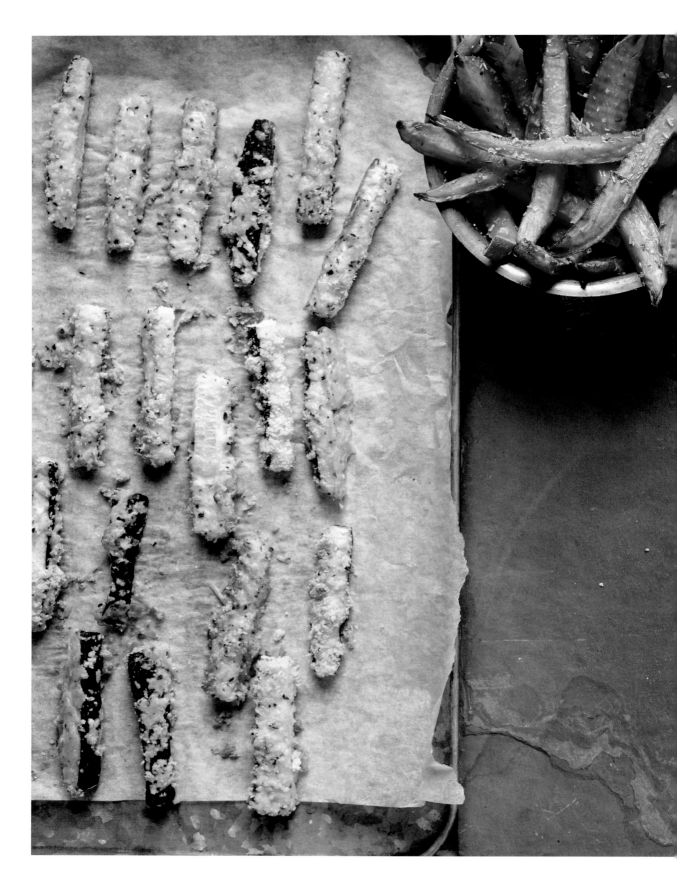

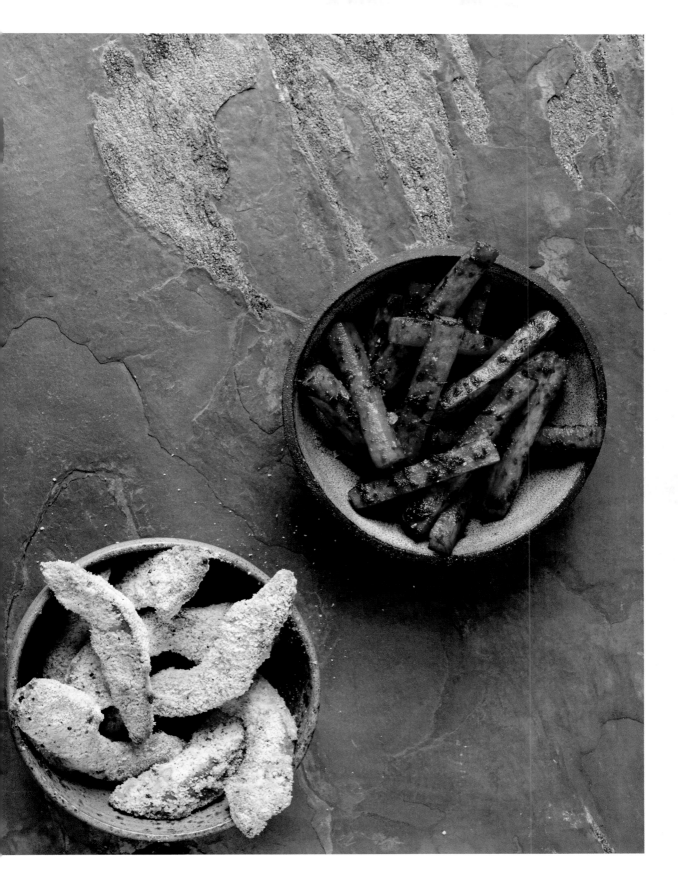

sesame kale crisps

Throw away that bag of carb-filled crisps and try these instead. Kale is green, healthy and perhaps not as appealing as your average bag of salted, fat-laden potato crisps; however, I can assure you that these are delicious, moreish and packed with flavour. They have the same crisp crunch as normal crisps but are blood sugar-friendly.

This recipe makes a bowl big enough to share among four people before supper, or to hand around at a picnic. I like to scatter a handful of them over a mixed salad at lunchtime.

 4   **5 MINS**   **9–11 MINS**

150g kale, tough stalks removed and leaves chopped into bite-sized pieces

1 tbsp tahini paste

2 tbsp olive oil

juice of ½ lemon

3 tbsp sesame seeds

1 tsp sea salt flakes

1. Preheat the oven to 200°C/400°F/gas mark 6 and line 2 baking sheets with greaseproof paper.

2. Put the kale in a large bowl and add the tahini, olive oil and lemon juice.

3. Massage the tahini, oil and lemon juice into the leaves with your hands until the leaves are all coated.

4. Sprinkle in the sesame seeds and toss the kale to evenly coat (you can keep a few back to sprinkle on top before placing in the oven, if you like).

5. Divide the kale between the baking sheets and spread the leaves out so that they aren't all on top of each other. Try to leave a little space between each kale leaf.

6. Sprinkle over the reserved sesame seeds (if you kept some back) and the sea salt.

7. Bake into the oven for 9–11 minutes, until the edges are browning very slightly and the kale is dark green (keep a close eye on the kale while it's cooking as it burns very quickly).

8. Remove from the oven and pop all the kale into a beautiful bowl to hand around!

NUTRITIONAL INFORMATION
(per serving)

Calories	Carbs
142.75	6.85g
Total Fat	**Protein**
12.49g	3.23g

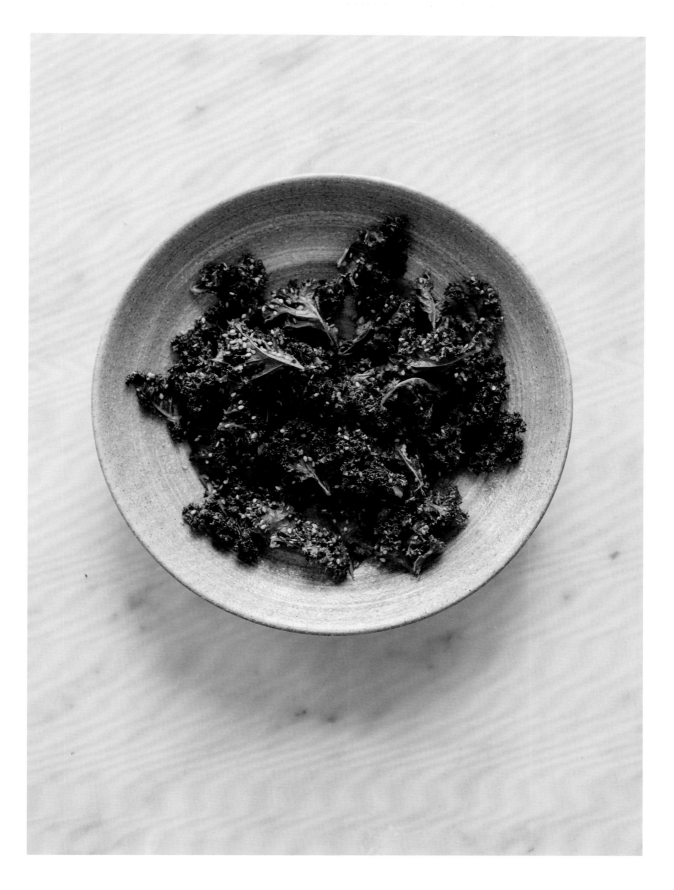

sea salt and lemon zest almonds

The perfect savoury snack, full of zing and crunch. This is a purse-string-friendly snack that you'll have nothing to feel guilty about and will be able to enjoy by the handful. The secret ingredient to this dish is egg white – it's what binds all the flavours to the almonds and helps give them the much-loved crunch.

 6   **5** MINS   **15–20** MINS, PLUS COOLING

1 large egg white

300g whole almonds

grated zest of 1 large lemon and 1 tbsp juice

pinch of sea salt flakes

1. Preheat the oven to 200°C/400°F/gas mark 6 and line a large baking sheet with baking parchment.

2. Place the egg white in a large, clean mixing bowl and whisk until it forms stiff peaks. Tip in all the almonds and coat them in the egg white. Add the lemon zest and juice and mix until fully combined.

3. Spread the almonds evenly over the baking sheet – bake them in two batches if necessary – and generously sprinkle over the sea salt.

4. Bake for 15–20 minutes until golden and toasted – keep a close eye on them after 15 minutes to check that they don't burn. You will hear them start to crackle when they are nearly done.

5. Remove from the oven very carefully as the nuts will be scorching hot, then leave to cool.

6. Once cooled, break them up, as they will be stuck together a little from the egg white, and place in an airtight container. They can be stored like this for up to 3 weeks.

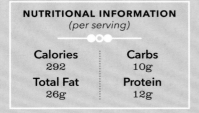

NUTRITIONAL INFORMATION
(per serving)

Calories	Carbs
292	10g
Total Fat	**Protein**
26g	12g

cracked pepper and sea salt multi-seed crackers

Delicious and simple, these grain-free multi-seed crackers make a low-carb savoury snack that is perfect for sharing, taking on the go or enjoying with some full-fat cheese. It always feels much more rewarding knowing that you've made something that's blood sugar-friendly. I like to eat mine with mashed avocado and roasted red onion slices.

 6   **15 MINS**   **20 MINS**

1 large egg

1 tbsp olive oil

140g ground almonds

160g mixed seeds (I use golden and brown linseed, pumpkin and sunflower seeds)

1 tsp cracked black pepper

½ tsp sea salt

1. Preheat the oven to 190°C/375°F/gas mark 5.

2. Beat the egg and olive oil in a mixing bowl until pale and combined. Mix in the ground almonds, mixed seeds, pepper and salt and combine to form a dough.

3. Place one sheet of baking parchment on a baking sheet and put the dough on top, then put another sheet over it to cover. Press the dough down slightly, then roll it out into a flat square with a rolling pin. It needs to be about 5mm thick. Remove the top layer of baking parchment and set it aside for later use.

4. Cut off the ragged edges of the dough but keep the bits, as you can roll them out again and make a few more biscuits.

5. Carefully score the dough with a sharp knife to make 9–12 even-sized squares, but don't cut all the way through. Repeat with the remaining dough (if you have any offcuts).

6. Place the baking sheet in the oven and cook for 20 minutes until the crackers are golden brown. When you remove them from the oven do not be alarmed if there is a little foam on top: this will evaporate almost straightaway.

7. Once cooled, the biscuits will break away from each other very easily and can be eaten immediately or stored in an airtight container for up to 10 days.

NUTRITIONAL INFORMATION
(per serving)

Calories	Carbs
322	10g
Total Fat	**Protein**
29g	13g

chia and chocolate orange energy balls

Energy balls are everywhere these days and, although they all look and sound delicious, they are usually filled with dried fruits, which make them very high in carbs and sugars.

These energy balls are very low in carbs, have a wonderful brownie-like consistency, a deep aroma of chocolate and tangy orange taste.

 MAKES 14   **10 MINS**   **1 HOUR**

120g almond butter

25g coconut oil, melted

50g unsweetened
 desiccated coconut

2 tbsp unsweetened cocoa
 powder

grated zest of 1 medium
 orange and 1 tbsp juice

2 tbsp chia seeds

50g ground almonds

1. Put the almond butter, coconut oil and desiccated coconut in a high-powered blender or food processor and blitz for 1–2 minutes until well combined, thick and creamy. Add the cocoa, orange zest and juice, chia seeds and ground almonds and blitz again for about 2 minutes until fully combined and sticky. If it does not stick together well, blitz for a little longer.

2. Taking a tablespoon of the mixture and mould it into a ball with your hands. Place each ball on a plate and repeat until you have used up all the mixture.

3. Place the plate of balls in the freezer for 1 hour, covered, until well set.

4. Remove and keep in a sealed container in the fridge for up to 2 weeks. Alternatively, keep in the freezer in a sealed container for up to 3 months.

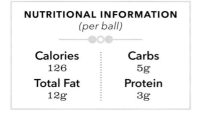

NUTRITIONAL INFORMATION
(per ball)

Calories	Carbs
126	5g
Total Fat	**Protein**
12g	3g

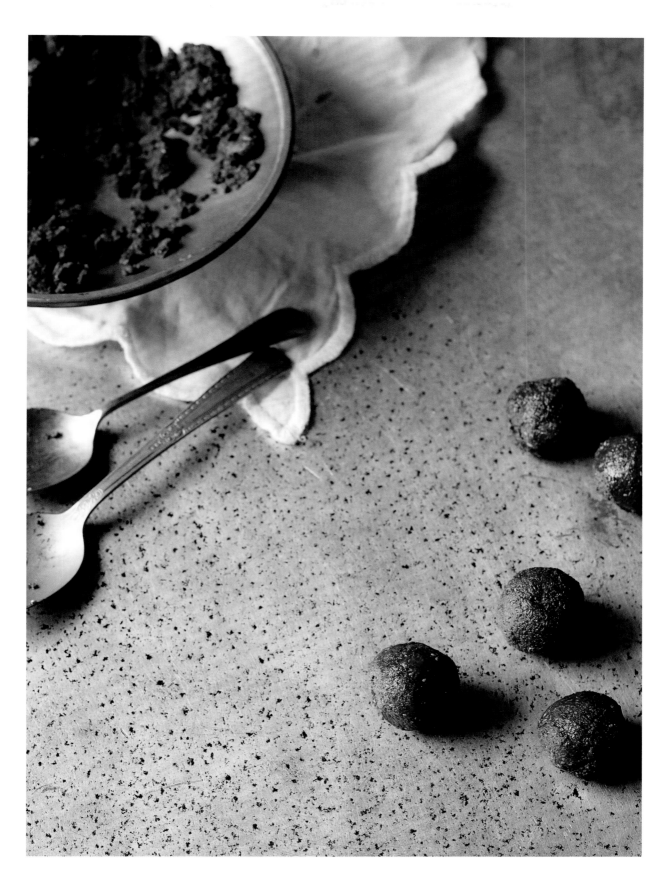

peanut butter cups

A simple, homemade, two-ingredient treat. These are incredibly indulgent, yet not full of sugar, with a delicious shell of chocolate and a smooth peanut butter centre. Always use the highest-percentage cocoa-content chocolate you can find, and the best quality. If you cannot eat peanut butter, substitute with another nut butter or seed butter of choice.

 MAKES 12 **10 MINS** **50 MINS**

125g dark chocolate
(85 per cent cocoa solids),
broken into pieces

4½ tbsp smooth peanut
butter

NOTES: Using a lower cocoa percentage chocolate will increase the carb and sugar content.

   If the peanut butter is not completely smooth, add a little melted coconut oil to it and stir until smooth.

   To make mini peanut butter cups, use 24 mini muffin paper cases: perfect for taking on the go and more kid-friendly than larger cups.

1. Line a 12-cup cupcake tin with paper cases.

2. Melt the chocolate in a glass bowl over a small pan of simmering water, stirring regularly, making sure the bottom of the bowl doesn't touch the water. Remove from the heat and add 1½ tablespoons of the peanut butter. Mix well until combined.

3. Pour a little of the chocolate/peanut mixture (about 1½ teaspoons) into the bottom of each paper case, then place them in the freezer for 20 minutes until solid.

4. Remove from the freezer and divide the remaining peanut butter evenly among the centres of each chocolate cup until you have used it all up.

5. Pour the remaining chocolate/peanut mix evenly into each cup and place back in the freezer for a further 30 minutes until solid.

6. Remove from the freezer and store in a sealed container in the fridge for up to 10 days. Serve chilled or allow to sit at room temperature for 10–15 minutes for a softer texture.

7. You can decorate the top with cacao nibs, grated orange zest, chilli flakes or some grated dried coconut to jazz them up a little, without adding more carbs!

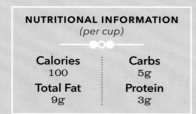

NUTRITIONAL INFORMATION
(per cup)

Calories	Carbs
100	5g
Total Fat	**Protein**
9g	3g

chocolate coconut cups

These chocolate coconut cups are divine and will curb any craving you might have for a sweet treat. They are incredibly simple to make and combine the luxuriously creamy consistency of coconut with deep, dark and intensely flavoured fine dark chocolate.

Perfect for sharing or keeping in a sealed container in the fridge to delve into as and when you want a guilt-free taste of decadence.

 MAKES 16   **15 MINS**   **40–55 MINS**

For the base

25g coconut oil, plus extra for greasing (if needed)

130g unsweetened desiccated coconut

35ml coconut milk

For the topping

150g dark chocolate (85 per cent cocoa solids), broken into pieces

Optional toppings

½ tsp toasted coconut flakes per cup

a pinch of dried chilli flakes on each cup

4 cacao nibs per cup

1 tsp chopped nuts per cup

½ tsp mixed seeds per cup

1. Grease 16 holes in a few muffin tins or fill them with paper cases.

2. Melt the coconut oil in a small saucepan over low heat.

3. Blitz the desiccated coconut, coconut milk and melted coconut oil on high speed in a food processor for 1 minute until the mixture is sticky. If you don't have a food processor, remove the coconut oil from heat and stir in the shredded coconut and coconut milk until the mixture is combined and sticky.

4. Divide the mixture evenly among each paper case, pressing firmly with your fingers or the back of a spoon to help them stick together. Place the tins in the freezer for 20–30 minutes, or until the coconut cups have hardened.

5. Just before the end of the freezing time, heat the chocolate in a glass bowl over a small pan of simmering water, stirring regularly (making sure the bottom of the bowl doesn't touch the water), until melted and smooth.

6. Spoon about 1 tablespoon of melted chocolate onto each coconut bite. If using any of the optional toppings, sprinkle them on immediately after spooning over the melted chocolate as the chocolate will harden quickly.

7. Place the tins back in the freezer for 20–25 minutes or until the chocolate coconut cups are fully set. Gently remove the cups from the tin and enjoy, or store in an airtight container in the fridge for up to 10 days.

NOTE: The higher the percentage of cocoa solids in chocolate, the lower the carb content. If you find 85 per cent too bitter, opt for 70 per cent, but be aware that each serving will have a higher sugar content.

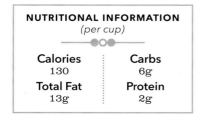

NUTRITIONAL INFORMATION
(per cup)

Calories	Carbs
130	6g
Total Fat	**Protein**
13g	2g

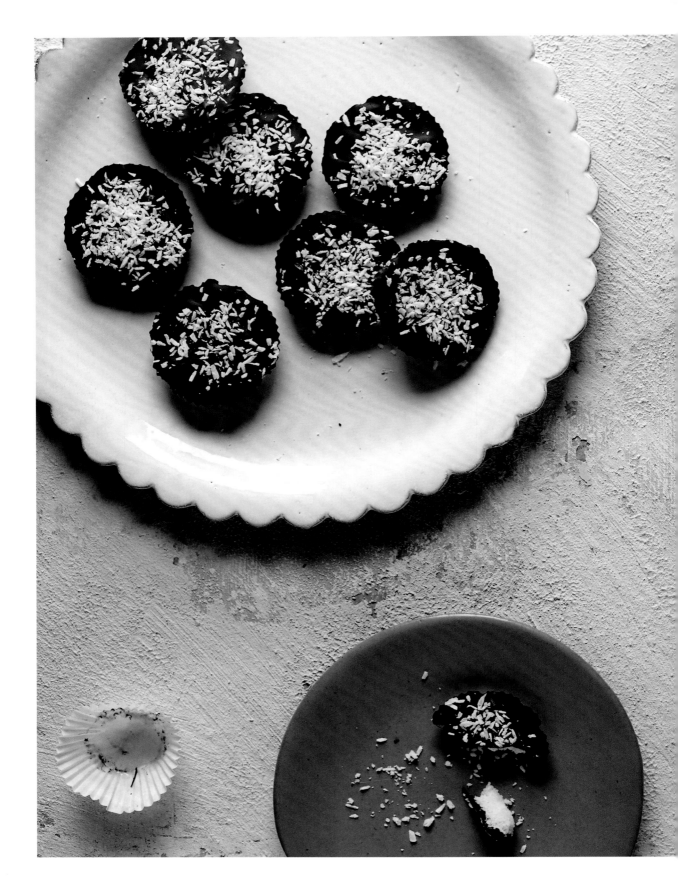

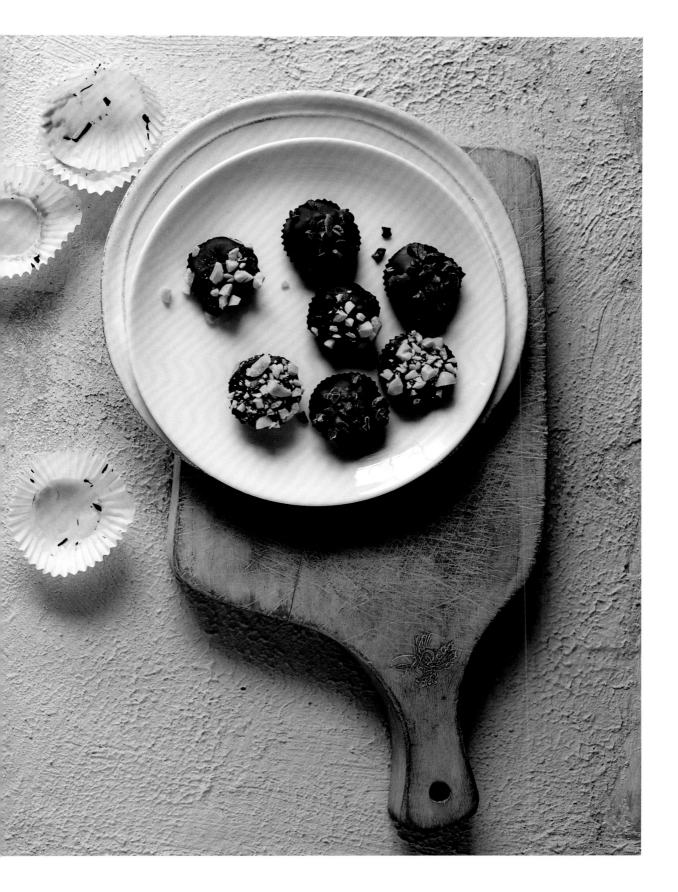

chocolate shortbread squares

These chocolate shortbread squares are divine: they require no baking whatsoever and are very low in carbs. The thick chocolate topping with the shortbread base is a beautiful combination of tastes and textures. If I'm on the go I like to take a couple with me so that I don't find myself reaching for anything I shouldn't. They curb any sweet cravings without sending my blood sugar levels sky high.

The cashew nut butter gives a slightly sweet taste without adding sugar or carbs and really does bring out the flavour of shortbread. If you'd like to add some flavours to the chocolate topping, there are some suggestions below.

 MAKES 12   **15 MINS, PLUS STANDING**   **1 HOUR**

100g ground almonds

100g unsweetened desiccated coconut

2 tbsp cashew nut butter

a pinch of sea salt

100g dark chocolate (85 per cent cocoa solids), broken into pieces

1 tbsp coconut oil

VARIATIONS:

○ Add 1 tsp grated orange zest to the chocolate mixture with 2 tbsp flaked almonds for a delicious zing and crunch.

○ Add ½ tsp peppermint extract to the chocolate mixture.

○ Sprinkle ½ tsp grated lemon zest and 1 tbsp goji berries on top for a vibrant decoration.

1. Blitz the ground almonds, coconut, cashew nut butter and sea salt in a food processor for about 2 minutes until sticky and bound together. You might have to scrape down the sides a couple of times.

2. Press the mixture into a silicone mould or a greased brownie dish to form a flat base. I like to keep mine about 1cm thick, but you can have it as thin or thick as you want. Place in the freezer for about 30 minutes until solid.

3. Melt the chocolate and coconut oil in a glass bowl over a small pan of simmering water, stirring regularly, making sure the bottom of the bowl doesn't touch the water. Pour the chocolate directly onto the shortbread base and place in freezer for a further 30 minutes or until set.

4. Remove from the freezer and allow to stand for 15–20 minutes, then use a sharp knife to cut it into squares. Dip the knife blade into boiling water first to heat and it should cut through without any difficulty.

5. Keep the squares in a sealed container in the fridge for up to 10 days.

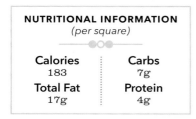

NUTRITIONAL INFORMATION	
(per square)	
Calories	Carbs
183	7g
Total Fat	Protein
17g	4g

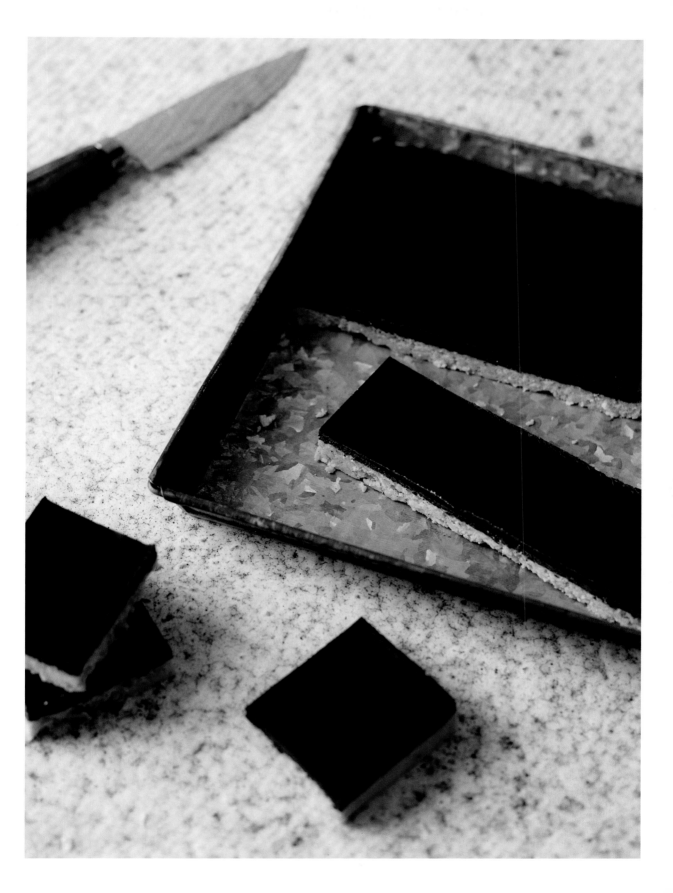

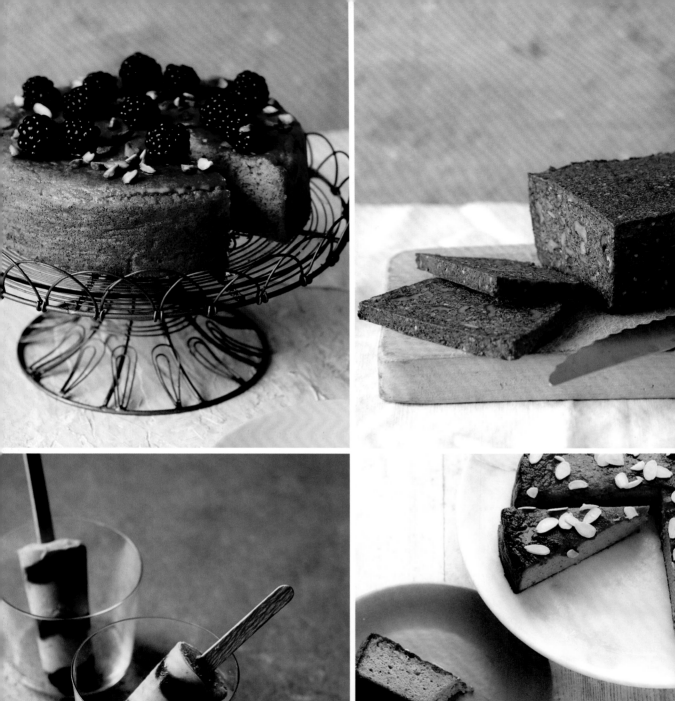
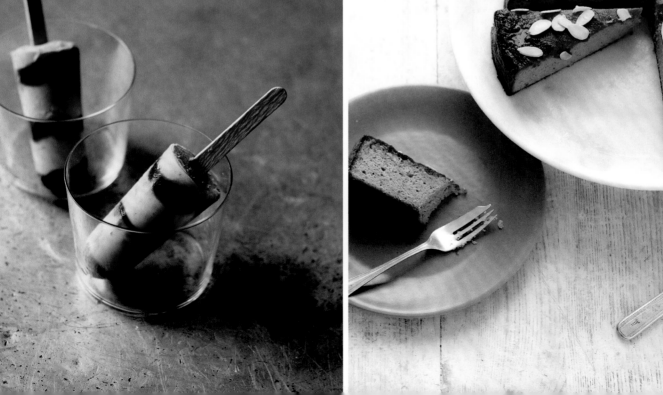

Baking & desserts

super seed bread

One thing that people miss more than anything when following a low-carb lifestyle is bread. This grain-free recipe is foolproof, I guarantee. It has a similar consistency to rye bread, can be toasted and has a good flavour, which most non-wheat breads do not. It doesn't crumble, tastes delicious, has a crust and will last for up to a week – although I can assure you that it will be consumed long before then.

It doesn't rise like normal bread, so it isn't as 'tall' as your usual shop-bought loaf. My favourite way to eat it is toasted with mashed avocado, sea salt flakes and a soft-boiled egg on top. Or, if I fancy something a little sweeter, I have a thicker slice slathered with Hazelnut chocolate spread (see page 71). However you choose to enjoy it, it will become a firm favourite, I promise!

 MAKES 1 LOAF (ABOUT 18 SLICES)   **10 MINS**   **1 HOUR**

300g mixed seeds (the choice is yours; I use flax, sunflower and pumpkin, poppy seeds, etc.)

100g ground almonds

50g chia seeds

50g walnuts or other type of nut, chopped

½ tsp grated nutmeg

1 tsp each sea salt and cracked black pepper

3 large eggs, beaten

1. Preheat the oven to 200°C/400°F/gas mark 6.

2. First, grind 200g of the mixed seeds: place the seeds in a high-powered blender or coffee grinder and blitz on high speed until they have a flour-like consistency.

3. Put the ground seeds in a large bowl with the remaining mixed seeds, ground almonds, chia seeds, walnuts, nutmeg, salt and pepper and combine with a spoon. Create a well and add the beaten eggs, then stir until fully combined. Add 200ml water and combine until you have a thick mixture.

4. Transfer the batter to a 900g loaf tin (I use silicone, but if you use an alternative, make sure it's greased) and bake in the oven for 1 hour until the top is golden and a skewer inserted into the middle of the loaf comes out clean, checking it after 40 minutes and covering the top with foil to prevent it burning, if necessary.

5. Remove from the oven and allow to cool fully before serving. It will keep in an airtight container for up to a week.

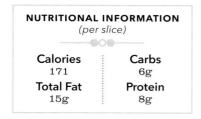

NUTRITIONAL INFORMATION (per slice)	
Calories 171	Carbs 6g
Total Fat 15g	Protein 8g

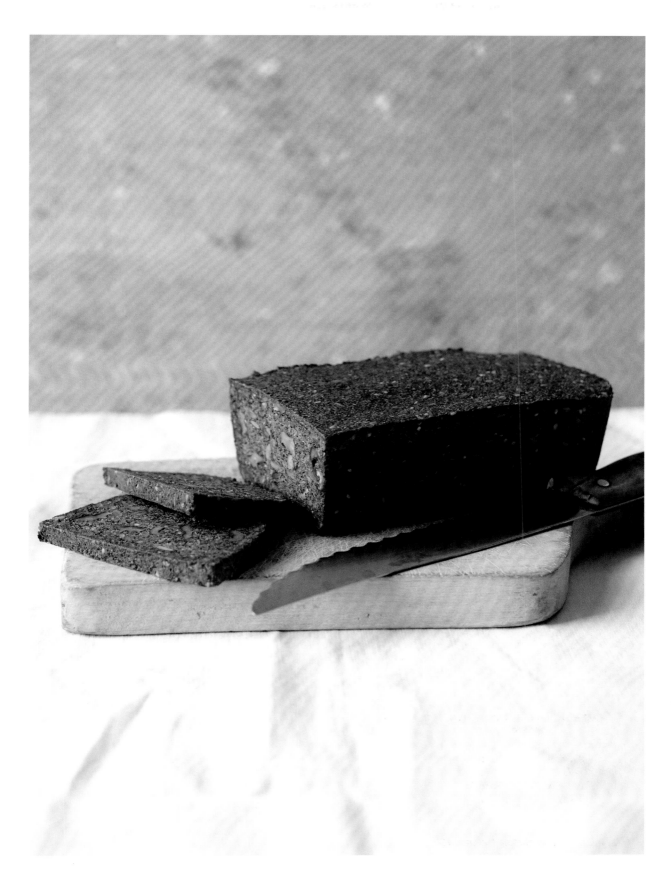

breakfast loaf

A beautiful bread that's naturally sweet, packed with the subtle spices of cinnamon and nutmeg and the added warmth of ginger. It's great eaten freshly sliced, or toasted and generously slathered with butter. The sweet potato and goji berries give it all the sweetness it needs and make it the perfect breakfast loaf.

Of course, this isn't your usual springy white loaf. It has a similar consistency to rye bread, but on the plus side, it isn't packed full of carbs.

 Makes 1 loaf (18–20 slices)   **15 mins**   **1 hour**

250g sweet potatoes, peeled

200g whole or ground seeds such as linseed, pumpkin, sunflower (you can use any you like so long as the total adds up to 200g)

30g goji berries

30g chia seeds

50g ground almonds

1 tsp ground cinnamon

1 tsp ground ginger

¼ tsp grated nutmeg

3 large eggs, beaten

a handful of seeds, for sprinkling

1. Preheat the oven to 200°C/400°F/gas mark 6.

2. Grate the sweet potato across the medium-sized holes of a box grater or use a food processor with the grating function. Put it in a clean tea towel and squeeze out any excess moisture. Set aside.

3. Place the whole seeds and goji berries in a food processor and blitz until they are finely ground and resemble flour. If you are using ground seeds, just blitz the goji berries.

4. Combine all the dry ingredients – the ground seeds and goji berries, chia seeds, ground almonds, cinnamon, ginger and nutmeg – in a large bowl. Make a well in the dry ingredients and stir in the beaten eggs, 90ml water and the grated sweet potato until well combined. Leave to stand for 5 minutes, to allow the chia seeds to soak up some of the moisture.

5. Transfer the batter to a 900g loaf tin (I use silicone, but if you use an alternative, make sure it's greased) and spread it out evenly.

6. Sprinkle a handful of seeds on top, then place the tin in the centre of the oven and bake for about 1 hour, or until the top is golden and a skewer inserted into the centre of the loaf comes out clean, checking it after 40 minutes and covering the top with foil to prevent it burning, if necessary.

7. Remove from the oven and allow to cool fully before serving. It will keep in an airtight container for up to a week.

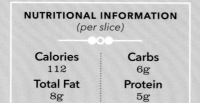

NUTRITIONAL INFORMATION
(per slice)

Calories	Carbs
112	6g
Total Fat	**Protein**
8g	5g

banana bread

This is a loaf for the whole family. Sweetened only with bananas, it's a simple, moist and textured loaf that's filling and flavour-packed. I have made this recipe on countless occasions, especially since weaning my daughter as she absolutely adores bananas so they are always piled high in the fruit bowl, ripening at a speed of knots – the riper the banana, the better the banana bread! Use very ripe bananas as they are naturally sweeter, give added moisture to the bread and bake beautifully.

Bananas are high in carbs so be aware of this when slicing.

 MAKES 1 LOAF (16 SLICES)   **15 MINS**   **45 MINS**

4 ripe bananas (about 500g)

4 large eggs, beaten

50g coconut oil, melted

1½ tsp ground cinnamon

80g ground almonds

20g coconut flour

1 tsp baking powder

80g walnuts, chopped (optional)

1. Preheat the oven to 200°C/400°F/gas mark 6.

2. Put 450g of the banana in a food processor with the eggs (chop the other 50g banana into slices to decorate the top), and blitz until creamy and combined.

3. Carefully add in the melted coconut oil, continuing to blend the mixture. Add the cinnamon, ground almonds, coconut flour and baking powder and blitz again.

4. Transfer the batter to a bowl and stir in the chopped walnuts, if using.

5. Pour the batter into a 900g loaf tin (I use silicone, but if you use an alternative, make sure it's greased) and spread it out evenly, then decorate the top with the chopped banana.

6. Bake in the oven for 45 minutes. Check the bread is cooked through by inserting a skewer into the centre of the cake and seeing if it comes out clean – it might seem a little bubbly from the coconut oil but this will solidify as the bread cools.

NOTE: If you don't have a food processor, mash the banana by hand to a smooth consistency, then add all the other ingredients as per the steps above.

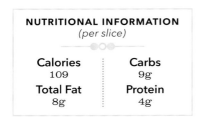

NUTRITIONAL INFORMATION (per slice)	
Calories 109	Carbs 9g
Total Fat 8g	Protein 4g

blackberry and pistachio cake

This is one of my all-time favourite cake recipes; it has an incredibly indulgent, moist texture, with the delicious combination of sweetness and the tartness of blackberries. It's the perfect summer cake to be enjoyed outside in the sunshine with a big pot of tea when the blackberry season is in full swing.

This cake is lower in carbs per slice than your average sugar-filled shop-bought cake, but please be mindful that the suggested serving is one slice per person. I usually serve it with a big dollop of crème fraîche.

 MAKES 1 CAKE (12 SLICES)   **15 MINS**   **50 MINS**

butter or oil, for greasing

100g shelled pistachio nuts

6 large eggs, separated

200g ground almonds

80g muscovado sugar or coconut sugar

125g blackberries, plus extra to decorate

a small handful of chopped shelled pistachios, to decorate

1. Preheat the oven to 200°C/400°F/gas mark 6 and grease and line a 20cm diameter round cake tin.

2. Put three-quarters of the pistachio nuts in a blender and blitz until they have a flour-like consistency. Add the egg yolks, ground almonds and sugar and blitz for 20–30 seconds until fully combined. Transfer to a mixing bowl.

3. In a clean, large bowl, whisk the egg whites until they form stiff peaks.

4. Gently fold the egg whites into the pistachio mixture with a metal spoon until fully combined, then fold in the blackberries and remaining pistachio nuts (I chop mine up a bit first) and transfer to the cake tin.

5. Pop in the oven for about 50 minutes until a skewer inserted into the middle of the cake comes out clean. Transfer to a wire rack to cool in the tin, then turn out to cool fully.

6. Decorate the cake with chopped pistachios and blackberries.

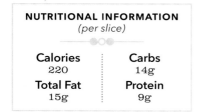

NUTRITIONAL INFORMATION
(per slice)

Calories	Carbs
220	14g
Total Fat	**Protein**
15g	9g

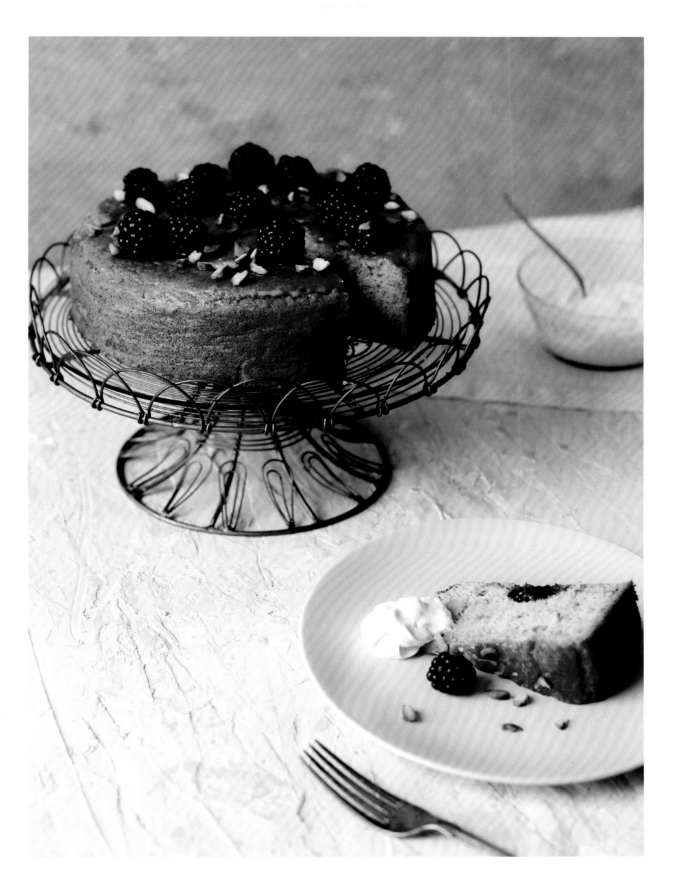

orange and almond cake

Everyone deserves a treat now and then, diabetes or not. The important thing is knowing what you are eating and always being mindful about carbs and sugar. With just four key ingredients, this is a cake you will end up making again and again. As far as cakes go, this is fresh, moist, aromatic, moreish and incredibly easy to make. Being completely grain and dairy free means the carb content is naturally much lower than that of a normal cake, too, though it is still a cake and so should only really be enjoyed for special occasions – hard as it might be, restrict yourself to one slice.

 MAKES 1 LARGE CAKE (16 SLICES)   **20 MINS**   **3 HOURS, PLUS COOLING**

For the cake
2 large oranges

240g almond flour

250g coconut palm sugar

a pinch of sea salt (optional)

6 large eggs, separated

To finish
2 tbsp flaked almonds

1 tsp coconut oil

1. Put the whole oranges in a large pan of boiling water and boil for 10 minutes then reduce the heat and simmer for about 1 hour 50 minutes until the skins are tender and the oranges feel soft. Drain and allow to cool for 30 minutes.

2. Preheat the oven to 200°C/400°F/gas mark 6.

3. Over a bowl, remove the pips from the boiled oranges and put the skin, juice and orange flesh in a blender with the flour, sugar and salt, if using. Blitz, then add the egg yolks and blitz until smooth. Transfer to a large bowl.

4. In a separate, large clean bowl, whisk the egg whites until they form stiff peaks then fold them into the orange mixture and gently combine.

5. Pour the cake batter into a 23cm non-stick springform round cake tin and bake for about 1 hour. Check the cake after about 40 minutes; if the top is browning too much, cover it with foil. Insert a skewer into the middle of the cake – if it comes out clean it's ready. Transfer to a wire rack to cool in the tin, then turn out to cool fully.

6. While the cake cools, dry-toast the flaked almonds in a pan over high heat until golden brown. Tip onto a plate and set aside. Melt the coconut oil in a pan, then pour into a small pot or jug and cool for 2–3 minutes. Once the cake has fully cooled, pour the glaze over the cake and decorate with the almonds.

7. Store in a sealed container in the fridge for up to 5 days.

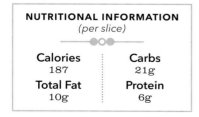

NUTRITIONAL INFORMATION *(per slice)*	
Calories 187	Carbs 21g
Total Fat 10g	Protein 6g

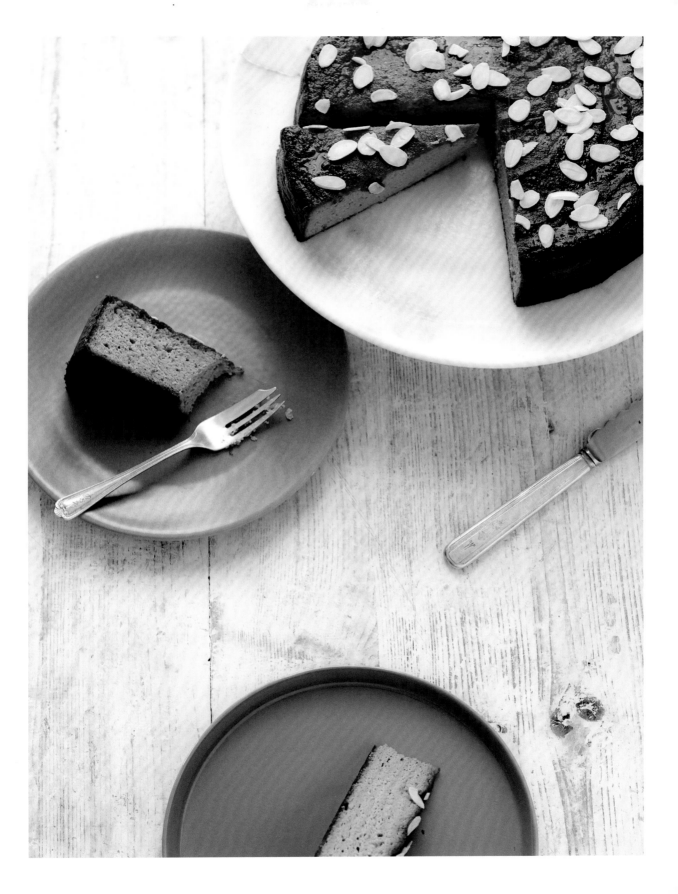

apple and cinnamon muffins

Divine, moist, filling, buttery, tasty and moreish are just a few of the many comments that are made about this recipe. They are simple and straightforward to make and the whole family will love them. Full of warm, spicy cinnamon and delicious apple pieces, they are perfect enjoyed straight from the oven, for breakfast, afternoon tea or as a snack on the go. The baking aroma alone will leave guests begging you for the recipe. Use whatever apple you prefer: I like to use Braeburn, Gala, Granny Smith or Pink Lady.

 MAKES 8   **20 MINS**   **25 MINS**

150g ground almonds

2 tsp ground cinnamon

½ tsp ground ginger

2 large eggs, beaten, at room temperature

80g butter, melted

200g apples, peeled, cored and cut into small cubes

1. Preheat the oven to 200°C/400°F/gas mark 6 and line a 12-hole muffin tin with 8 muffin cases.

2. In a medium bowl, mix together the ground almonds, cinnamon and ginger.

3. In a large bowl, beat together the eggs and melted butter.

4. Add the dry mix to the wet and stir until thick and combined, then gently fold in the chopped apples.

5. Divide the batter evenly among the muffin cases, filling them almost full.

6. Bake for 25 minutes until risen, with a firm golden top, or until a skewer inserted in the middle of one of the muffins comes out clean.

7. Let the muffins cool for 5 minutes in the tin, then transfer to a wire rack to cool.

8. Store in an airtight container at room temperature for 1 day or in the fridge for up to 3 days.

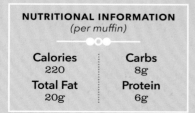

NUTRITIONAL INFORMATION
(per muffin)

Calories	Carbs
220	8g
Total Fat	**Protein**
20g	6g

apple pie

This twist on the classic apple pie has a thick, spice-infused, grain-free pastry base and a tart apple filling and is perfect to slice and share. It holds together beautifully and is as delicious straight from the oven as it is served up cold three days later. Serve with a generous dollop of full-fat crème fraîche, Greek yoghurt or a teaspoon of clotted cream.

 10   **25 MINS**   **30 MINS**

For the crust

200g ground almonds

60g coconut flour

20g unsweetened desiccated coconut

1 tsp ground cinnamon

¼ tsp grated nutmeg

1 tsp ground ginger

1 large egg, beaten, plus 1 yolk, for the pie glaze

20g butter or coconut oil, melted, plus extra for greasing

For the apple filling

5 large cooking apples (about 900g), peeled, cored and cubed

1 tsp ground cinnamon

750ml water

½ tbsp coconut oil

NOTE: The pie keeps well in an airtight container for up to a week, or frozen for up to 3 months.

NUTRITIONAL INFORMATION	
(per slice)	
Calories	Carbs
220	21g
Total Fat	Protein
15g	7g

1. Preheat the oven to 200°C/400°F/gas mark 6. Lightly grease a 22cm round pie dish and set aside.

2. Put the ground almonds, coconut flour, desiccated coconut, cinnamon, nutmeg and ginger in a large bowl and mix to combine. Add the beaten egg and stir together to form a crumbly mixture. Drizzle in the melted butter or coconut oil, stirring to combine. Add 30ml water, little by little, continuing to stir, until the mixture holds together, then use your hands to form it into a ball of dough. If the mixture feels too dry, add a little more water.

3. Put three-quarters of the dough into the pie dish and press it in evenly with your fingers. Line the pastry with greaseproof paper, add baking beans and blind bake for 13–15 minutes or until the crust is very lightly browned.

4. While the crust is baking, make the filling. Put the apples, cinnamon and water in a pan. Bring to the boil over high heat, then cover, reduce the heat and simmer, stirring occasionally, for 30 minutes, or until the apples are soft and the water has evaporated.

5. While the apples are cooking, roll out the remaining dough between two sheets of greaseproof paper, then cut into lattice strips or shapes with a sharp knife.

6. Remove the apples from the heat and stir in the coconut oil. Mash the apple to a smoother consistency.

7. Remove the greaseproof paper and baking beans from the blind-baked pie crust and spoon in the apple mixture. Place the dough strips or shapes on top, brush the crust with egg yolk and bake for 15 minutes until the filling is bubbling and the crust is golden brown. Remove and allow to cool for about 15 minutes before serving.

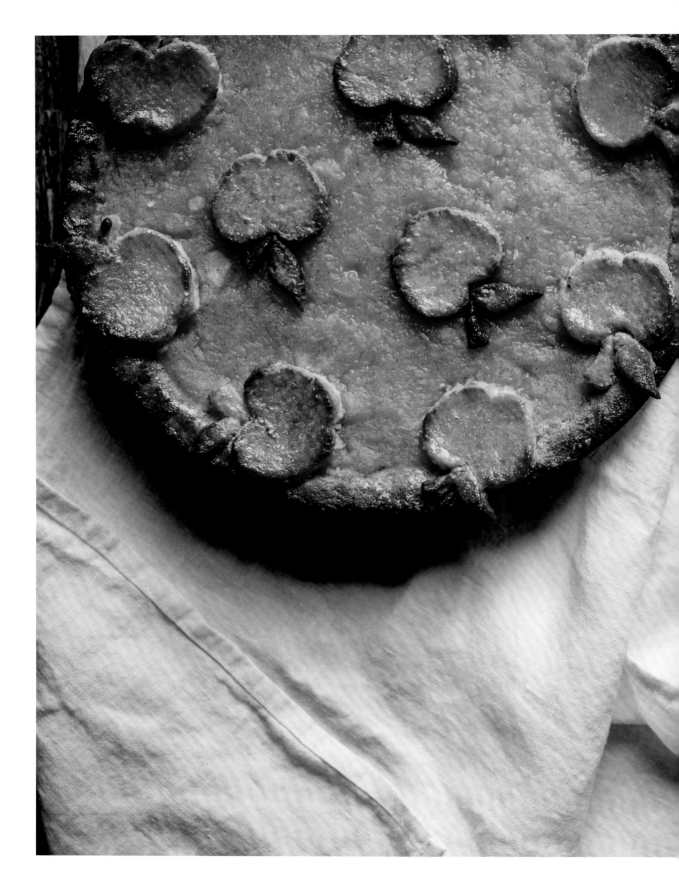

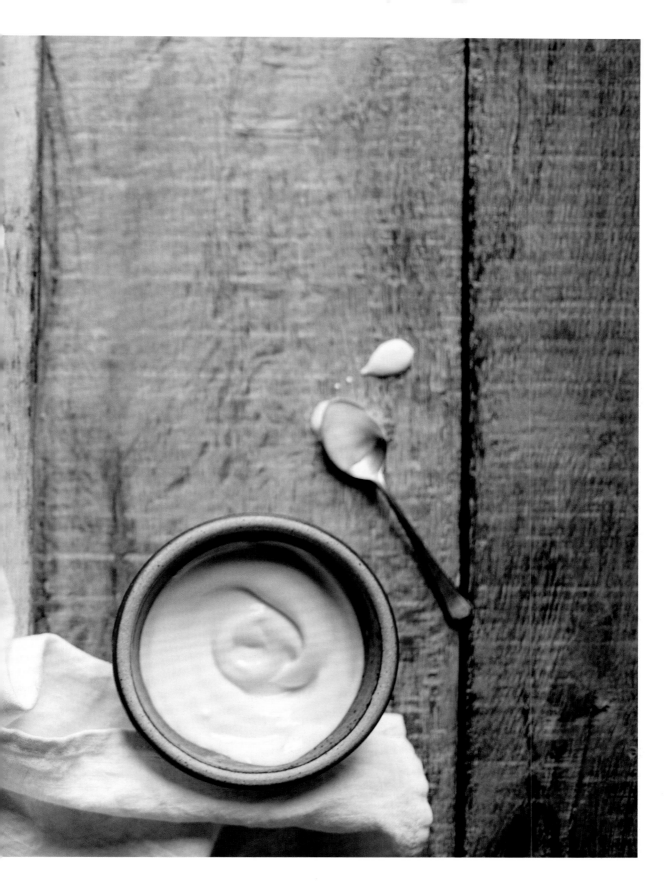

light chocolate orange pots

This is an incredibly indulgent, creamy chocolate mousse. It is perfect for rounding off a feast with family or friends. It takes just minutes to make but needs a little forward-planning as the coconut milk needs to sit in the fridge overnight and the mousse requires at least five hours to set. You only need small portions as it has an intense flavour. If you think it will taste too 'coconutty', think again – this recipe has been tested on many people and no one has ever identified coconut as an ingredient. Try to use coconut milk that only contains the milk itself and water, avoiding those with additives. Serve with a dollop of crème fraîche and chopped, toasted hazelnuts.

 4   **15 MINS** **OVERNIGHT FOR COCONUT MILK, PLUS AT LEAST 5 HOURS TO SET**

1 x 400g tin full-fat coconut milk

80g dark chocolate (85 per cent cocoa solids), broken into pieces

1 tsp grated orange zest

1. Pop the tin of coconut milk in the fridge overnight.

2. Remove the tin from the fridge and do not shake it. Open the tin and scoop out the coconut cream which will have separated from the liquid and settled at the top of the tin. Pop it into a bowl. You need 150g of coconut cream, so if you have less add some of the water from the tin. Whisk together well. Discard the remaining coconut liquid.

3. Fill a small pan with 5cm depth of water and bring to the boil over high heat. Reduce to a simmer, then carefully place a heatproof bowl over the pan and add the chocolate pieces and melt for a minute or two, stirring regularly. Once melted, remove the bowl from the pan.

4. Add the coconut cream, whisking regularly until fully combined. You will notice that the mixture will turn from a light brown colour to a deeper brown and thicken as you whisk.

5. Stir in the orange zest and thoroughly combine.

6. Place equal-sized servings of the chocolate mixture into 4 small ramekins or small pots and pop into the fridge to set for at least 5 hours.

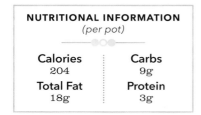

NUTRITIONAL INFORMATION
(per pot)

Calories	Carbs
204	9g
Total Fat	**Protein**
18g	3g

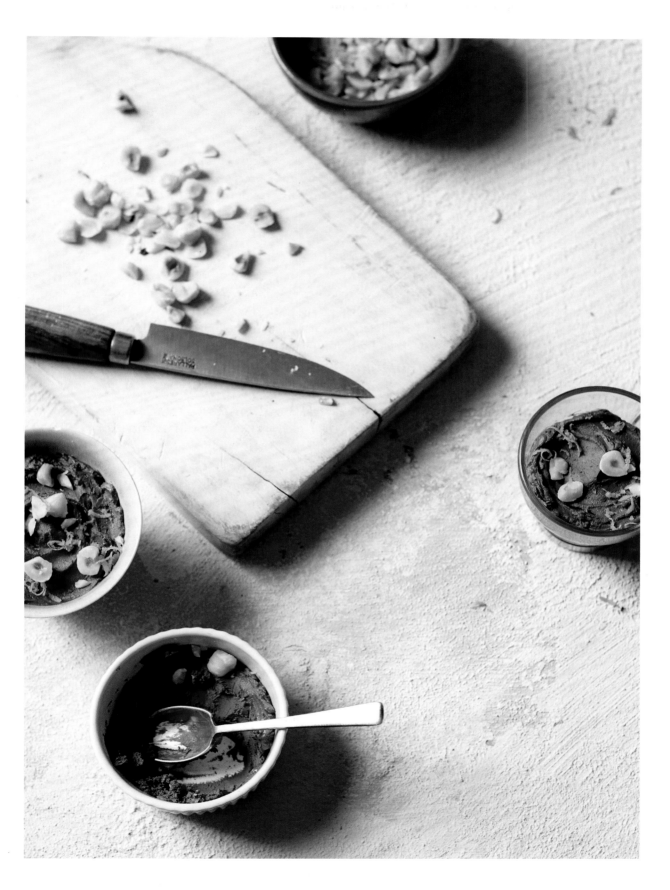

cherry, chocolate and coconut cream ice lollies

This might seem like a blazingly obvious recipe, but sometimes the simplest ingredients make for the most wonderful flavours. These lollies are all about getting the right balance between the sweetness of the cherries, the full-bodied cocoa taste and the creaminess of the Greek yoghurt.

Cherries are in season for such a short amount of time that it's crucial we embrace and enjoy them as much as possible. The darker and riper the cherry, the sweeter it is. Cherries, of course, do contain carbs, but as far as fruits go they are on the lower end of the carb scale.

 MAKES 6   **10 MINS**   **6 HOURS**

300g cherries (pre-stoned weight)
60g full-fat Greek yoghurt
50g 85 per cent plain chocolate, broken into pieces

1. Remove all the stones from the cherries. Place the flesh from the cherries into a high-powered blender and blitz on high to a dark, thick, smoothie-like consistency.

2. Add the Greek yoghurt and pulse a few times until fully combined.

3. Pour equal amounts among 6 lolly moulds, then pop a stick into each one, carefully cover with cling film and put in the freezer for at least 6 hours or until solid and frozen through.

4. Place a small pan over medium heat with about 5cm of water in it. Bring to the boil, then reduce to a simmer before carefully placing a glass bowl on top (so that it fits safely but doesn't touch the water). Put the chocolate in the bowl and heat for a minute or two until melted, stirring regularly. Set aside.

5. To remove the lollies from their moulds, fill a bowl with warm water and dip the lolly moulds into it for about 1 minute. The lollies should then slide out.

6. Place the lollies on a sheet of greaseproof paper and drizzle the melted chocolate all over them.

7. Once the melted chocolate has set, transfer to a sealed container and keep in the freezer until required.

NOTE: You could also add chopped nuts when you drizzle with chocolate if you want to add something extra.

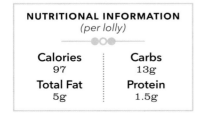

NUTRITIONAL INFORMATION	
(per lolly)	
Calories	Carbs
97	13g
Total Fat	Protein
5g	1.5g

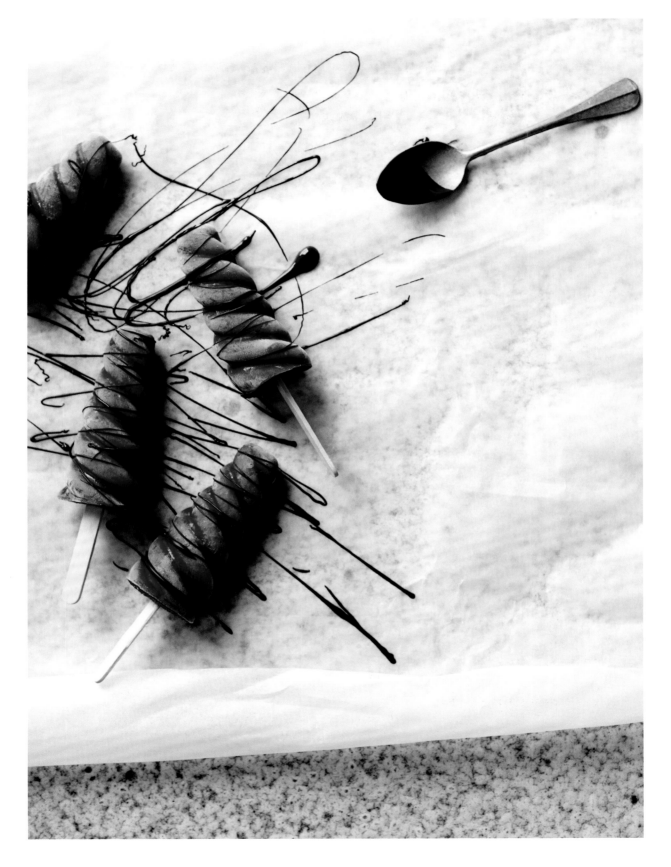

blueberry and Greek yoghurt ice lollies

A refreshing, fruity, low-carb, blood sugar-friendly treat. The perfect blend of fruit and cream. These lollies are great for munching in the garden, as a sweet treat after work or as an alternative to the jingle-jangle from the ice-cream van.

They are good for the whole family and completely guilt free, so put that sugary ice-cream cone down, grab your blender and get creative. Not only will your body thank you for it, but so will anyone you share them with.

 MAKES 6   20 MINS   6 HOURS

165g blueberries
50ml water
550g full-fat Greek yoghurt (if you are dairy free, use a 400ml tin coconut milk)

1. Place the blueberries into a small pan over high heat with the water. Gently bring to the boil, then reduce to a simmer.

2. Cook for about 10 minutes until the blueberries have softened and the skins have started to peel away. Mash them gently with a spoon to break them down.

3. Continue to stir until all the water has evaporated and the coulis has started to thicken. Set aside to cool.

4. Place 2 tablespoons of the blueberry coulis into a blender with the Greek yoghurt and blitz for a few seconds until smooth and creamy.

5. Gently pour the coulis into the bottom of 6 lolly moulds, then top up with a layer of blueberry cream. Continue this process until all mixture has been used in each lolly mould (you can be as creative as you like with layering the mixtures).

6. Place the lollipop sticks gently into the mix before covering carefully with cling film and popping into the freezer for at least 6 hours.

7. Keep in the freezer until ready to serve!

NOTE: Try making different swirls and shades by mixing more or less blueberry coulis with the yoghurt.

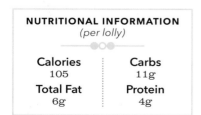

NUTRITIONAL INFORMATION
(per lolly)

Calories	Carbs
105	11g
Total Fat	**Protein**
6g	4g

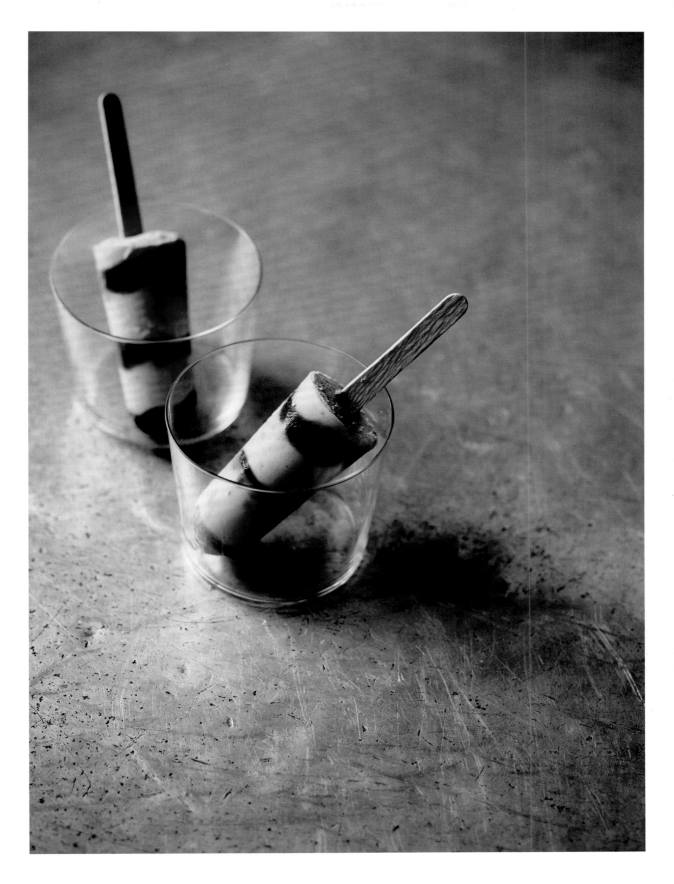

Meal Planners

In order to help you keep your blood glucose under control we have prepared two weeks of meal planners, one lower in carbs and one higher. The carbs and calories have been worked out per person, per meal, per day. We have added a low-carb and a higher-carb option to give you the flexibility to mix and match the meals to fit around your family and lifestyle.

Creating meal plans for yourself is a great way of effectively managing your daily carbohydrate intake, giving you more variety, monitoring your portion control and avoiding those unnecessarily sugary and calorific impulse buys.

LOW-CARB MEAL PLANNER

	MONDAY	TUESDAY	WEDNESDAY	THURSDAY
BREAKFAST	Spinach, sun-dried tomato and goat's cheese omelette (p37) *Carbs: 8g, Calories: 430*	2 English breakfast muffins (p54) *Carbs: 2g, Calories: 138*	Greek yoghurt with blueberry and lime jam and toasted seeds (p63) *Carbs: 11g, Calories: 164*	Baked breakfast mushrooms (p45) *Carbs: 4g, Calories: 143*
LUNCH	Scotch egg with crunchy nut crust (p110) *Carbs: 9g, Calories: 672*	Roasted aubergine and garlic salad with olive oil, basil and tomato (p86) *Carbs: 14g, Calories: 329*	Courgette 'spaghetti' with pesto and chicken (p94) *Carbs: 13g, Calories: 433*	Tomato, basil and mozzarella salad with pan-fried mackerel (p100) *Carbs: 6g, Calories: 537* Chocolate and shortbread square (p194) *Carbs: 7g, Calories: 183*
DINNER	Almond butter chicken curry with cauliflower rice (p133) *Carbs: 24g, Calories: 422*	Egg-fried cauliflower rice with chicken (p136) *Carbs: 18g, Calories: 411*	Mixed fish skewers with a spicy nut butter dip (p104) *Carbs: 15g, Calories: 383*	Coconut chicken nuggets with tomato and sweet paprika sauce (p144) *Carbs: 14g, Calories: 660*
TOTAL DAILY CARB (G)	41	34	39	31

Friday	SATURDAY	SUNDAY
One-pan bacon, eggs and asparagus (p38) *Carbs: 2g, Calories: 107*	Baked eggs in avocado with roasted fennel and tomatoes (p44) *Carbs: 12g, Calories: 291*	Zesty lime, courgette and spring onion fritters (p50) *Carbs: 8g, Calories: 248*
Beetroot and coconut soup (p76) *Carbs: 25g, Calories: 302*	Pesto and Parma ham pizza (p108) *Carbs: 9g, Calories: 311* Peanut butter cup (p190) *Carbs: 5g, Calories: 100*	Sausage, red onion, sun-dried tomato and spinach frittata (p52) *Carbs: 12g, Calories: 345*
Brilliant beef burgers (p151) *Carbs: 12g, Calories: 587*	Creamy cashew chicken with tarragon and lemon (p134) *Carbs: 15g, Calories: 542*	Stuffed turkey breast with garlic, nuts and olives (p146) *Carbs: 10g, Calories: 385* Smoky carrot fries (p180) *Carbs: 4g, Calories: 78*
39	**41**	**34**

Green vegetables such as spinach, kale and broccoli are all nutritious, low-carb additions to a meal and are very versatile. They can be stir-fried, roasted, steamed or eaten raw. To increase the level of antioxidants and vitamins consumed during a meal try eating a handful of berries such as blueberries and a few nuts after the main dish.

Handful of wild rocket
    Carbs: 1.5g, Calories: 8

½ avocado, sliced
    Carbs: 6g, Calories: 130

50g broccoli and 70g kale,
    stir-fried in a little butter
    Carbs: 10g, Calories: 135

30g fresh spinach with ½ avocado,
    drizzled with olive oil
    Carbs: 7g, Calories: 256

Side salad of 3 cherry tomatoes,
    10 black olives and a handful of rocket
    Carbs: 6g, Calories: 54

50g steamed broccoli
    Carbs: 6g, Calories: 28

Handful of raspberries (about 10)
    Carbs: 2, Calories: 10

Handful of blueberries
    Carbs: 3g, Calories: 11

100g Greek yoghurt (plain)
    Carbs: 6g, Calories: 120

Handful of almonds (about 12)
    Carbs: 3g, Calories: 85

Handful of pumpkin seeds (30g)
    Carbs: 1g, Calories: 190

HIGHER-CARB MEAL PLANNER

	MONDAY	TUESDAY	WEDNESDAY	THURSDAY
BREAKFAST	Sweet potato and kale rosti with baked eggs (p40) *Carbs: 22g, Calories:181*	Mixed berry mini muffin omelettes (p55) *Carbs: 5g, Calories: 195*	Cinnamon pancakes with Greek yoghurt (p62) *Carbs: 21g, Calories: 622*	Sausage, red onion, sun-dried tomato and spinach frittata (p52) *Carbs: 12g, Calories:345*
LUNCH	Roasted Mediterranean vegetable couscous (p90) *Carbs: 16g, Calories: 93* Cheesy courgette fries (p181) *Carbs: 4g, Calories: 196*	Pea and bacon soup (p82) *Carbs: 22g, Calories: 302*	Peppered paprika salmon (p97) *Carbs: 4g, Calories: 451* Homemade coleslaw (p96) *Carbs: 10g, Calories: 77*	Butternut, feta and Tenderstem salad with tahini and toasted seeds (p84) *Carbs: 23g, Calories: 260*
DINNER	Nutty mushroom risotto with bacon (p150) *Carbs: 21g, Calories: 339*	Baked cod with a pistachio pesto crust (p156) *Carbs: 9g, Calories: 444* Blueberry and Greek yoghurt ice lolly (p214) *Carbs: 10g, Calories: 105*	Roasted aubergine with kale pesto (p163) *Carbs: 19g, Calories: 331*	Cheesy cauliflower pizza (ham, fig and rocket) (pp166–7) *Carbs: 19g, Calories: 293*
TOTAL DAILY CARB (G)	63	46	54	54

FRIDAY	SATURDAY	SUNDAY
sweet potato, leek and lime fritter (p51) *Carbs: 13g, Calories: 99*	Crushed avocado toast with soft-boiled egg and bacon (p42) *Carbs: 15g, Calories: 484*	Sweet potato, green cabbage and red onion hash with fried peppered eggs (p46) *Carbs: 16g, Calories: 186*
Courgette 'spaghetti' with pesto and chicken (p94) *Carbs: 13g, Calories: 433*	Baked chicken tikka pieces (p106) *Carbs: 11g, Calories: 308* Garlic and rosemary sweet potato fries (p180) *Carbs: 15g, Calories: 123*	Creamy mushroom soup (p79) *Carbs: 13g, Calories: 206*
Mrs P's cottage pie (p152) *Carbs: 22g, Calories: 447* Crushed creamy peas with basil (p174) *Carbs: 7g, Calories: 68*	Fiery steak stir-fry with spinach, pine nuts, onion and garlic (p154) *Carbs: 16g, Calories:579* Peanut butter cup (p190) *Carbs: 5g, Calories: 100*	Coconut chicken tikka (p132) *Carbs: 14g, Calories: 330* Cauliflower rice (p133) *Carbs: 11, Calories: 89*
55	**62**	**53**

See page 217 for suggested side dishes and snacks.

Index

Page references in *italics* indicate images.

Acknowledgements

With great thanks to my baby girl, Florence, my most treasured sous chef, and to my husband, Ports, for trying my failures and my successes, and always being honest and believing in me. Heartfelt thanks also to my ever-supportive, loving parents.

A special thanks to David Cavan: it has been a huge honour to work on this book with him and a privilege to have his trust, support and belief in my recipes.

Thanks to my agent, Jonathan Hayden, whose hard work and dedication made this book possible; and also to Jules Gammond, Henrique Coimbra, Amy Picanco, Lara Clarke, Melanie Houghton, Simon Cope, Amy, Will and Elowen Searle, Rob and Tess Porter; to my brilliant diabetes team at Great Western Hospital, most notably Amanda Martin; to the wonderful creative work of Laura Nickoll, Sophie Yamamoto, Kim Lightbody and Becci Woods; and to PRH for believing in our vision.

And that leaves me with my wonderful readers, who have stuck with me throughout my journey from blogger to author! Diabetes is a hard disease, it is 24/7, 365 days a year. There is so much support out there for everyone with diabetes and their families, especially from online communities and forums such as diabetes.co.uk. Be open, honest, ask questions and never forget that you control your diabetes, it shouldn't control you.
Emma Porter

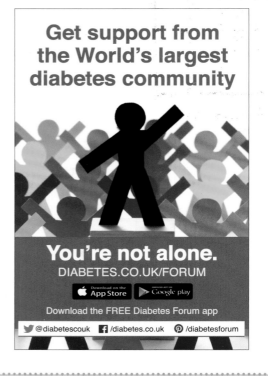

I am hugely grateful to Emma, whose passion, determination and adaptability as well as her skill as a creator of great recipes, made this book possible.
David Cavan